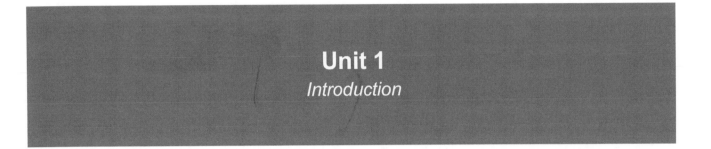

Unit 1
Introduction

Introduction to Medical Word Building

Learning Objective

This module teaches medical word building, including root words, combining forms, prefixes, and suffixes.

Medical terminology is likely the most difficult and extensive written section of your training. Throughout this course and in medical transcription editing, you will be exposed to what may be an entirely new vocabulary, totally foreign to your experience.

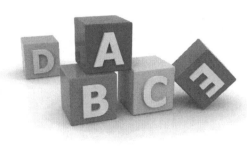

English medical terms are primarily adopted from the Latin and Greek languages, and this makes learning these terms much like learning a new language. The good news is that because of this, medical terminology follows relatively consistent language rules, which should help you assimilate the terms. This module breaks down the terms into their respective word parts, i.e., prefixes, suffixes, and root words, and teaches how to combine them. By learning these pieces and the rules for combining them, you will be able to create literally thousands of new medical words.

When you see a word you are unfamiliar with, it makes sense to stop and look up the definition of the word. You should also, when able, listen to the pronunciation of unfamiliar words. Many online dictionaries have pronunciation tools, and the training program has a pronunciation tool as well.

If you have previously studied terminology in college courses, such as premed, nursing, or terminology classes, you should find that experience especially helpful in this section.

Of course, focusing on terminology and learning these terms will enhance your ability to recognize medical words when they are dictated and when you are performing the actual medical transcription editing. You may have noticed in prior modules that most of the sentences used as examples and in exercise work have been medically oriented and contained words unfamiliar to you. The next several units will introduce you to a variety of medical words from all medical specialties.

It is important to remember as you proceed through the units in this module that never in an actual transcription or editing setting will you be required to translate from the English definition of a medical term to its proper medical form. In other words, dictators will not require you to "put in a word that means profuse sweating" as they dictate. They will always use the appropriate medical term (in this case, *diaphoresis*) and you will only be expected to hear it and then spell it correctly in the report. Therefore, as you go through the exercises in this module, recognize that there will occasionally be word parts that share the same English meaning, and you will want to choose the one that is found more recently in the coursework, and pat yourself on the back for realizing that more than one is possible.

Every student enrolled in the Career Step Medical Transcription Editing Program receives a **15-month** subscription to Benchmark KB (Knowledge Base) online, the industry's first application designed to increase the quality and speed of medical transcription and transcription editing through the use of health data standards. BenchMark KB is a complete set of web services that brings together an extensive collection of online medical transcription/editing reference materials into a single application, with real time updates to keep students up to date on terminology and reference data.

Keep your resources (Benchmark KB, hard copy, etc.) handy as you work through Medical Word Building. You will find that sometimes more than one prefix or suffix is a possible acceptable answer. For example, if you are told to come up with a word that means "inside the cranium," you can choose intracranial, endocranial, or encranial since "intra," "endo," and "end" all mean "inside of" or "within." **The only way to be sure that you have a bona fide word is to check in a reputable resource and see if it is there.** In the example cited, you will find both "intracranial" and "endocranial." The only definition for "endocranial" is "intracranial," so you know that "intracranial" is the preferred form. What adjectival ending is the proper one? What noun ending is the most commonly used one? Which prefix is correct? The only way to tell is to make liberal use of your resources.

Learning these definitions will be a tremendous aid to your ability to distinguish and locate the appropriate terms when you hear them dictated in medical reports. Do not try to rush through the exercises, however. There is a lot of new material and information, and you should give your mind time to assimilate it.

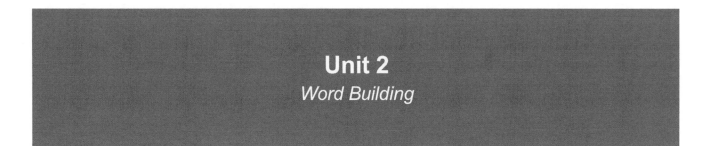

Unit 2
Word Building

Word Structure – Introduction

This first unit will teach you the different word parts and how to combine them accurately. As you may know, most medical words have Latin and Greek origins. Although at first medical terms may seem complicated and perhaps impossible to learn, they are made up of prefixes, suffixes, and root words which are relatively limited in number and quite easy to learn. You will thus first learn word parts; your knowledge of these parts and combining forms and your ability to recognize them will enable you to build an extensive medical vocabulary.

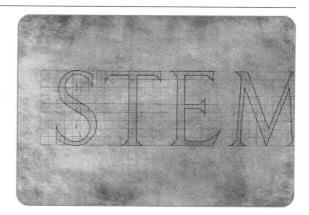

There are root words, prefixes, and suffixes. We'll begin with root words.

Root Word or Stem: *This is the main body or foundation of the word.*

Every word has at least one root, but a word can have two, three, or four. Any word containing more than one root word is known as a **compound** word. The English language has many compound words and one can make thousands of compound combinations. These occur often in everyday speech, and you are already familiar with many compound words. For example: crosswalk, everyday, milkman, storefront, backhoe, moonlighter, sidewalk, sidewinder, etc. In true compound words, both segments can stand alone as words. See the previous examples (cross, walk, every, day, store, front, etc.). Many medical words are also of this type: lymphadenopathy (lymph + adenopathy). You can thumb through your word list or any medical dictionary and see dozens of examples.

Combining Forms: *A combining form is a root plus a vowel.*

When creating words with the different word parts, the combining form plays a key role. The use of the vowel that makes up the combining form depends upon the vowel/consonant combination.

It is important when learning root words to also learn the combining vowels or vowel-consonant combinations that link them to other word parts. These vowels are **essential** to medical word building, as they are required between roots and other roots and suffixes to make appropriate compound words or words with suffix endings. In most cases, this makes it much easier to pronounce the words.

bronchospasm
Root Word: bronch
Combining Form: broncho
Suffix: -spasm

The combining vowel is necessary to create the word *bronchospasm*. It is difficult to pronounce bronchspasm in English.

Prefixes

A prefix is a syllable or syllables placed before a root word or compound word to modify it or give it new meaning.

Prefixes are not uncommon. In fact, you use them all the time. Some examples are pre- (as in prefix), re- (rerun), in- (insure), etc. In medical word building, prefixes are important. When prefixes are written alone they are followed by a hyphen, indicating that they require placement before another word (e.g., "pre- and postoperatively"). However, words with prefixes are one word and are **not** hyphenated.

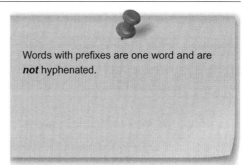

Words with prefixes are one word and are **not** hyphenated.

I. **FILL IN THE BLANK.**
    Determine the prefix in the following words and enter it in the blank provided.

1. preconceive _____   2. subcontract _____

3. bicycle _____   4. undress _____

5. bypass _____   6. implant _____

7. midabdomen _____   8. disconnect _____

9. transpose _____   10. preview _____

11. maladjusted _____   12. nonspecific _____

Suffixes

These are placed at the end of a word to modify it or to change its meaning.

These are also familiar to you. Some commonly used ones are -ment (advancement), -ance (resistance), -ness (kindness). As with prefixes, suffixes are a vital part of medical terminology. You should be able to determine what a suffix is and recognize it as familiar in an otherwise unfamiliar word.

I. **FILL IN THE BLANK.**
    Determine the suffix in the following words and enter it in the blank provided.

1. speculation_____   2. employment_____

3. dictionary_____   4. acceptable_____

5. rapidly_____   6. nervous_____

7. painful _____

8. remarkable _____

9. abdominal _____

10. receiver _____

Combining Forms

Remember, the definition of a combining form is "a root word plus a combining vowel." It is imperative to memorize the vowel that accompanies each root word, as you will need it to create many words. There are a few rules that govern word building.

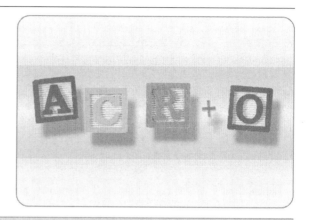

Rule 1: **The combining vowel is** *used when another* **root or suffix is added to the combining form and the added root word or suffix begins with a consonant.**

hepat/o + megaly = hepatomegaly
root word + combining form + suffix
hepat/o + splen/o + megaly = hepatosplenomegaly

Rule 2: **The combining vowel is** *dropped when the root word or suffix added to the combining form* **begins with a vowel.**

hepat/o + itis = hepatitis
root word + suffix

Rule 3: **Words that end in certain letters, most notably "x," substitute a "c" when combined with suffixes or plural endings.**

cervix + -al = cervical
thorax + -ic = thoracic

Rule 4: **Many prefixes end in a vowel and can be added to a root word or combining form without change to either. Any exceptions to this rule will be noted as they occur.**

I. **FILL IN THE BLANK.**
    Combine the following word parts. This is to test your comprehension of the word building rules. Don't worry about definitions; just apply the above rules.

    1. cyst/o + -cele _____

    2. amni/o + -centesis _____

    3. chol/e + cyst/o + -ectomy _____

    4. path/o + -logist _____

    5. bronch/o + spasm _____

    6. aden/o + pathy _____

    7. jejun/o + -ostomy _____

    8. ophthalm/o + -ic _____

    9. cervic/o + -itis _____

    10. salping/o + -ectomy _____

    11. col/o + -ostomy _____

    12. thorac/o + lumb/o + -ar _____

Identifying Word Parts

Now that you are able to combine various word parts, it is time to begin learning what they mean and how to spell them. The easiest way to learn a large number of medical terms in the shortest amount of time is to learn the various word parts. These, along with your knowledge of how to combine word parts, will give you the advantage of being able to create and/or identify thousands of medical terms.

I. **MATCHING.**
    Match the definitions to the following terms. Enter only the letter in the space provided (no punctuation).

    1. ____ root word

    2. ____ prefix

    3. ____ suffix

    4. ____ combining form

    A. A root word plus a vowel.
    B. The main body or foundation of a word.
    C. Syllable(s) placed at the end of a word to modify or change the meaning of the word.
    D. Syllable(s) placed at the front of a word to modify or change the meaning of the word.

II. FILL IN THE BLANK.
Combine the following word parts.

1. hydr/o + salpinx _____

2. chol/e + cyst/o + -ectomy _____

3. organ/o + -megaly _____

4. hyster/o + salping/o + -gram _____

5. chol/e + doch/o + jejun/o + -ostomy _____

6. esophag/o + gastr/o + duoden/o + -scopy _____

7. end/o + -scopy _____

8. lymph/o + aden/o + -ectomy _____

9. appendic/o + -itis _____

10. lumb/o + sacr/o + -al _____

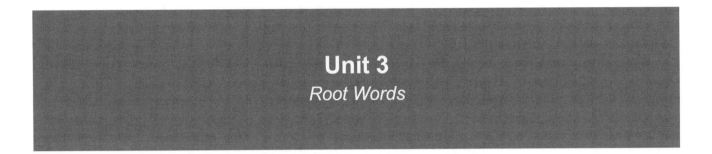

Unit 3
Root Words

Root Words – Introduction

This unit presents root words, or more accurately, combining forms (refer to the beginning of Medical Word Building for the difference). This category of word parts is by far the most extensive. These, along with prefixes and suffixes, are the building blocks for creating the extensive array of new medical words you are required to learn for transcription. Combining forms, as with the suffixes and prefixes, are arranged alphabetically. This unit covers root words A–X, as below.

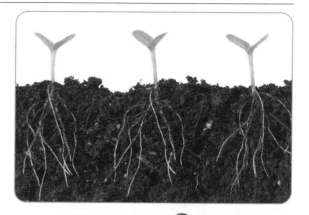

- *Root Words A–Ch in Lessons 1–8*
- *Root Words Ch–Ge in Lessons 9–16*
- *Root Words Ge–Me in Lessons 17–24*
- *Root Words Me–Pr in Lessons 25–32*
- *Root Words Ps–X in Lessons 33–41*

As a medical transcription editor, it is important to be able to recognize a root word when you hear it and combine it correctly with another combining form or different word part. Although it is not imperative that you know the exact meaning of every root word in the most technical sense, it is necessary that you be able to recognize and spell it correctly. You will also need to have at least a general idea of what the words mean to be sure that they make sense in context. Again, the more you know, the more valuable and efficient a medical transcription editor you are.

When you see a word you are unfamiliar with, it makes sense to stop and look up the definition of the word. You should also, when able, listen to the pronunciation of unfamiliar words. Many online dictionaries have pronunciation tools, and the training program has a pronunciation tool as well.

Without further ado, we will begin our study of root words with those beginning with the letters A–Ch.

Root Words – Lesson 1 (Ab–Ad)

Following is a list of combining forms with their accompanying meanings and a sample word. Memorize these combining forms for the subsequent exercises.

Word Part	Meaning	Example
abdomin/o	abdomen	abdominal
acr/o	extremities	acromegaly
aden/o	gland	adenocarcinoma
adenoid/o	adenoids	adenoidectomy
adip/o	fat	adipose

I. FILL IN THE BLANK.
Enter the words in the space provided.

1. abdominal _____   2. acromegaly _____

3. adenocarcinoma _____   4. adenoidectomy _____

5. adipose _____

II. MATCHING.
Match the appropriate terms below.

1. ____ acr/o
2. ____ aden/o
3. ____ abdomin/o
4. ____ adip/o
5. ____ adenoid/o

A. fat
B. gland
C. extremities
D. abdomen
E. adenoids

III. SPELLING.
Determine if the following words are spelled correctly. If the spelling is correct, leave the word as it has already been entered. If this spelling is incorrect, enter the word with the correct spelling.

1. adenoidectomy _____   2. adipoze _____

3. abdomenal _____   4. acromegaly _____

5. adnocarcinoma _____

Root Words – Lesson 2 (Ae–Am)

Following is a list of combining forms with their accompanying meanings and a sample word. Memorize these combining forms for the subsequent exercises.

Word Part	Meaning	Example
aer/o	air	aerobic
alb/o	white	albino
albumin/o	albumin	albuminemia
amni/o	amnion	amniotic
amyl/o	starch	amylase

I. FILL IN THE BLANK.
Enter the words in the space provided.

1. aerobic_____   2. albino_____

3. albuminemia_____   4. amniotic_____

5. amylase_____

II. MATCHING.
Match the appropriate terms below.

1. ____ albumin/o   A. white
2. ____ amni/o   B. air
                           C. starch
3. ____ amyl/o   D. albumin
4. ____ aer/o   E. amnion
5. ____ alb/o

III. MULTIPLE CHOICE.
Choose the appropriate answer for each.

1. Amylase indicates the presence of a (◯gas,◯starch).

2. The combining form aer/o means (◯air,◯evaporate).

3. The combining form in the word amniotic is (◯am/o,◯amni/o).

4. A person who is an albino is primarily affected by the color (◯black,◯white).

5. Amniotic tissue means it contains (◯amnion,◯amnien).

Root Words – Lesson 3 (An–Ap)

Following is a list of combining forms with their accompanying meanings and a sample word. Memorize these combining forms for the subsequent exercises.

Word Part	Meaning	Example
angi/o	vessel	angiogram
ankyl/o	crooked or fused	ankylosing
anter/o	anterior/before	anterolateral

| aort/o | aorta | aortic |
| append (ic) /o | appendix | appendicitis |

I. FILL IN THE BLANK.
Enter the words in the space provided.

1. angiogram_____

2. ankylosing_____

3. anterolateral_____

4. aortic_____

5. appendicitis_____

II. MATCHING.
Match the appropriate terms below.

1. ____ aort/o

2. ____ appendic/o

3. ____ anter/o

4. ____ ankyl/o

5. ____ angi/o

A. crooked
B. vessel
C. aorta
D. anterior
E. appendix

III. SPELLING.
Determine if the following words are spelled correctly. If the spelling is correct, leave the word as it has already been entered. If the spelling is incorrect, provide the correct spelling.

1. ankylosing _____

2. apendicitis _____

3. anteriolateral _____

4. aortec _____

5. angiogram _____

Root Words – Lesson 4 (Ar–At)

Following is a list of combining forms with their accompanying meanings and a sample word. Memorize these combining forms for the subsequent exercises.

Word Part	Meaning	Example
arteri/o	artery	arteriovenous
arthr/o	joint	arthroplasty
articul/o	joint	articulation
atel/o	imperfect	atelectasis
ather/o	yellow, fatty plaque	atheroma

I. FILL IN THE BLANK.
Enter the words in the space provided.

1. arteriovenous _____

2. arthroplasty _____

3. articulation _____

4. atelectasis _____

5. atheroma _____

II. MATCHING.
Match the appropriate terms below.

1. ____ articul/o

2. ____ ather/o

3. ____ atel/o

4. ____ arteri/o

5. ____ arthr/o

A. artery

B. joint

C. imperfect

D. yellow, fatty plaque

III. TRUE/FALSE.
Determine if the following statements are true or false. You need not be concerned with any suffixes you have not been exposed to at this point, as they will be presented in a future lesson.

1. Articulation involves a joint.
   ○ true
   ○ false

2. The word arteriovenous means there is no artery involved.
   ○ true
   ○ false

3. Arthroplasty involves a joint.
   ○ true
   ○ false

4. An atheroma involves purple plaque.
   ○ true
   ○ false

5. Atel/o means perfect.
   ○ true
   ○ false

Review: Lessons 1–4

I. MATCHING.
Match the appropriate terms below. Some terms may be used more than once.

1. ____ aden/o
2. ____ arthr/o
3. ____ anter/o
4. ____ aer/o
5. ____ ankyl/o
6. ____ acr/o
7. ____ aort/o
8. ____ articul/o
9. ____ amni/o
10. ____ abdomin/o
11. ____ angi/o
12. ____ alb/o
13. ____ amyl/o
14. ____ atel/o
15. ____ appendic/o
16. ____ adenoid/o
17. ____ adip/o
18. ____ albumin/o
19. ____ arteri/o
20. ____ ather/o

A. extremities
B. aorta
C. imperfect
D. abdomen
E. fat
F. yellow, fatty plaque
G. white
H. gland
I. starch
J. air
K. joint
L. crooked or fused
M. appendix
N. albumin
O. artery
P. amnion
Q. vessel
R. adenoids
S. anterior or before

II. MULTIPLE CHOICE.
You may need to do some research to answer the following questions, as you have not yet been exposed to some of the word combinations.

1. The word (○angiectomy, ○hematectomy) means excision of a blood vessel.

2. The word (○appendectomy, ○appendiceal) means excision of the appendix.

3. The word (○jointoplasty, ○arthroplasty) means surgical repair of a joint.

4. An (○arteriogram, ○arterioscope) would be a record of an artery.

5. The enzyme starch is written (◯amylase, ◯ezymylase).

6. Surgical excision of the adenoids is (◯adenectomy, ◯adenoidectomy).

7. The word (◯intra-abdominal, ◯interabdominal) means inside the abdomen.

8. The word (◯appendema, ◯appendicitis) means inflammation of the appendix.

9. The beginning or formation of fat is (◯adipogenesis, ◯albogenesis).

10. A word which means incision of the aorta is (◯aortectomy, ◯aortotomy).

Root Words – Lesson 5 (Au–Br)

Following is a list of combining forms with their accompanying meanings and a sample word. Memorize these combining forms for the subsequent exercises.

Word Part	Meaning	Example
aur/i	ear	auricle
bil/i	bile	biliary
blast/o	embryonic form	blastoma
blephar/o	eyelid	blepharitis
brachi/o	arm	brachiocephalic

I. **FILL IN THE BLANK.**
   Enter the words in the space provided.

1. auricle _____

2. biliary _____

3. blastoma _____

4. blepharitis _____

5. brachiocephalic _____

II. MATCHING.
Match the appropriate terms below.

1. ____ aur/i
2. ____ blephar/o
3. ____ blast/o
4. ____ brachi/o
5. ____ bil/i

A. bile
B. ear
C. arm
D. embryonic form
E. eyelid

III. MULTIPLE CHOICE.
Choose the correct answer.

1. The word auricle involves the (◯eye, ◯ear).

2. Blepharitis indicates the (◯eyelid, ◯earlobe) is involved.

3. Brachiocephalic indicates the (◯leg, ◯arm) is involved.

4. The combining form of blastoma is (◯bla/o, ◯blast/o).

5. The word (◯bile, ◯bill) is at the root of the word biliary.

Root Words – Lesson 6 (Br–Ca)

Following is a list of combining forms with their accompanying meanings and a sample word. Memorize these combining forms for the subsequent exercises.

Word Part	Meaning	Example
brachy	short	brachyesophagus
bronchi/o, bronch/o	windpipe	bronchospasm
bucc/o	cheek	buccal
burs/o	bursa	bursectomy
calc/i	calcium	calcification

I. FILL IN THE BLANK.
Enter the words in the space provided.

1. brachyesophagus _____

2. bronchospasm _____

3. buccal _____

4. bursectomy _____

5. calcification _____

II. MATCHING.
Match the appropriate terms below.

1. ____ bucc/o

2. ____ calc/i

3. ____ burs/o

4. ____ brachy

5. ____ bronchi/o

A. short
B. cheek
C. windpipe
D. calcium
E. bursa

III. SPELLING.
Determine if the following words are spelled correctly. If the spelling is correct, leave the word as it has already been entered. If this spelling is incorrect, enter the word with the correct spelling.

1. bronckospasm _____

2. buccal _____

3. brachyesofagus _____

4. bursectomy _____

5. calceum _____

Root Words – Lesson 7 (Ca)

Following is a list of combining forms with their accompanying meanings and a sample word. Memorize these combining forms for the subsequent exercises.

Word Part	Meaning	Example
calcane/o	heel	calcaneocuboid
carcin/o	cancer	carcinoma
cardi/o	heart	cardiomyopathy
carp/o	carpus/wrist	carpometacarpal
caud/o	tail	caudal

I. **FILL IN THE BLANK.**
   Enter the words in the space provided.

   1. calcaneocuboid _____

   2. carcinoma _____

   3. cardiomyopathy _____

   4. carpometacarpal _____

   5. caudal _____

II. **MATCHING.**
   Match the appropriate terms below.

   1. ____ cardi/o

   2. ____ carp/o

   3. ____ carcin/o

   4. ____ caud/o

   5. ____ calcane/o

   A. cancer
   B. tail
   C. heel
   D. heart
   E. carpus

III. **MISSING LETTERS.**
   In the following exercises there are letters missing from each term. Enter the completed term in the space provided.

   1. carc_no_a _____

   2. cardi_myop_thy _____

   3. cal_aneo_uboi_ _____

   4. c_rpo_etaca_pal _____

   5. c_rp_l _____

Root Words – Lesson 8 (Ce–Ch)

Following is a list of combining forms with their accompanying meanings and a sample word. Memorize these combining forms for the subsequent exercises.

Word Part	Meaning	Example
cec/o	cecum	cecal
cephal/o	head	cephalad
cerebr/o	brain	cerebral
cervic/o	neck	cervicothoracic
chlor/o	green	chlorophyll

I. FILL IN THE BLANK.
Enter the words in the space provided.

1. cecal_____   2. cephalad_____

3. cerebral_____   4. cervicothoracic_____

5. chlorophyll_____

II. MATCHING.
Match the appropriate terms below.

1. ____ cerebr/o   A. cecum
2. ____ chlor/o   B. head
                          C. brain
3. ____ cephal/o   D. green
4. ____ cervic/o   E. neck
5. ____ cec/o

III. TRUE/FALSE.
Determine if the following statements are true or false.

1. The word cephalad deals with the foot.
   ○ true
   ○ false

2. The word cerebral deals with the brain.
   ○ true
   ○ false

3. Chlorophyll indicates the color blue.
   ○ true
   ○ false

4. The word cervicalgia deals with the chest.
   ○ true
   ○ false

5. Cecal is correctly spelled in this sentence.
   ○ true
   ○ false

Review: Lessons 5–8

I. MATCHING.
Match the appropriate terms below.

1. ____ cardi/o
2. ____ bucc/o
3. ____ caud/o
4. ____ cervic/o
5. ____ blast/o
6. ____ burs/o
7. ____ carp/o
8. ____ cerebr/o
9. ____ aur/i
10. ____ blephar/o
11. ____ brachi/o
12. ____ calcane/o
13. ____ chlor/o
14. ____ carcin/o
15. ____ bil/i
16. ____ calc/i
17. ____ brachy
18. ____ cephal/o
19. ____ bronchi/o
20. ____ cec/o

A. ear
B. heart
C. eyelid
D. carpus
E. brain
F. head
G. cecum
H. embryonic form
I. cancerous
J. calcium
K. bursa
L. windpipe
M. short
N. tail
O. neck
P. heel
Q. green
R. arm
S. cheek
T. bile

II. MULTIPLE CHOICE.
You may need to do some research to answer the following questions, as you have not yet been exposed to some of the word combinations.

1. In a direction from head to tail is (◯cephalocaudal, ◯cephalotome) .

2. Pertaining to the ear is (◯aural, ◯oral) .

3. The hardening of a yellow, fatty plaque is (◯atheromatous, ◯atherosclerosis) .

4. Mucosa pertaining to the cheek would be (◯buckel, ◯buccal) mucosa.

5. Chronic dilatation of the windpipe is (◯bronchiectasis, ◯bronchyitis) .

6. A tumor in its embryonic form is (◯adnoidoma, ◯blastoma) .

7. Surgical excision of the cecum is (◯cecectomy, ◯cectomy) .

8. A cancerous tumor is (◯carcinoma, ◯carcinogenesis) .

9. Softening of the brain substance is (◯cephalomalacia, ◯cerebromalacia) .

10. Pain in the neck, radiating to the arm is (◯cervicobrachialgia, ◯radialgia) .

Root Words – Lesson 9 (Ch–Cl)

Following is a list of combining forms with their accompanying meanings and a sample word. Memorize these combining forms for the subsequent exercises.

Word Part	Meaning	Example
chol/e*	bile	cholecystectomy
cholecyst/o*	gallbladder	cholecystitis
chondr/o	cartilage	chondrocalcinosis
chori/o	fetal covering	chorioamnionitis
clavicul/o	clavicle	acromioclavicular

*Although 'chole' means bile, its most common usage is in the terms related to 'cholecyst' - gallbladder. The examples below use that term.

I. **FILL IN THE BLANK.**
   Enter the words in the space provided.

   1. cholecystectomy_____ 2. cholecystitis_____

   3. chondrocalcinosis_____ 4. chorioamnionitis_____

   5. acromioclavicular_____

II. MATCHING.
Match the appropriate terms below.

1. ___ chondr/o
2. ___ chori/o
3. ___ chol/e
4. ___ cholecyst/o
5. ___ clavicul/o

A. bile
B. cartilage
C. fetal covering
D. clavicle
E. gallbladder

III. MULTIPLE CHOICE.
Choose the appropriate answer for each.

1. A fetal covering is (◯chori/o,◯cholecyst/o).

2. Clavicul/o deals with the (◯cleft palate,◯clavicle).

3. Chondr/o deals with (◯cartilage,◯cranium).

4. Cholecyst/o means (◯gallbladder,◯liver).

5. Chol/e means (◯urine,◯bile).

Root Words – Lesson 10 (Co–Cr)

Following is a list of combining forms with their accompanying meanings and a sample word. Memorize these combining forms for the subsequent exercises.

Word Part	Meaning	Example
coccyg/o	coccyx	coccygeal
col/o	colon	colonoscopy
colp/o	hollow/vagina	colporrhaphy
cost/o	rib	costovertebral
crani/o	cranium/skull	craniocervical

I. FILL IN THE BLANK.
Enter the words in the space provided.

1. coccygeal _____

2. colonoscopy _____

3. colporrhaphy _____

4. costovertebral _____

5. craniocervical _____

II. MATCHING.
Match the appropriate terms below.

1. ____ col/o

2. ____ cost/o

3. ____ colp/o

4. ____ crani/o

5. ____ coccyg/o

A. hollow/vagina

B. coccyx

C. rib

D. colon

E. cranium/skull

III. SPELLING.
Determine if the following words are spelled correctly. If the spelling is correct, leave the word as it has already been entered. If this spelling is incorrect, enter the word with the correct spelling.

1. colinoscopy _____

2. cocygeal _____

3. craniocervical _____

4. costovertebril _____

5. colporhaphy _____

Root Words – Lesson 11 (Cr–Cy)

Following is a list of combining forms with their accompanying meanings and a sample word. Memorize these combining forms for the subsequent exercises.

Word Part	Meaning	Example
cry/o	cold	cryotherapy
crypt/o	hide, conceal	cryptogenic
cutane/o	skin	subcutaneous
cyan/o	blue	cyanosis
cyst/o	cyst, bladder	cystitis

I. FILL IN THE BLANK.
Enter the words in the space provided.

1. cryotherapy _____

2. cryptogenic _____

3. subcutaneous _____

4. cyanosis _____

5. cystitis _____

II. MATCHING.
Match the appropriate terms below.

1. ____ cutane/o

2. ____ cyst/o

3. ____ crypt/o

4. ____ cry/o

5. ____ cyan/o

A. cyst, bladder
B. cold
C. skin
D. hide, conceal
E. blue

III. FILL IN THE BLANK.
Enter the appropriate term in the space provided using the terms in this lesson.

1. The word part cry/o means _____.

2. The word part cutane/o deals with the _____.

3. Cyanosis indicates the color is _____.

4. A word part which means hide or conceal is _____.

5. A word part meaning bladder is _____.

Root Words – Lesson 12 (Cy–De)

Following is a list of combining forms with their accompanying meanings and a sample word. Memorize these combining forms for the subsequent exercises.

Word Part	Meaning	Example
cyt/o (-cyte)	cell	plasmacytoma
dactyl/o	finger, toe	hexadactylism
dent/i dent/o	teeth	dental
derm/a dermat/o	skin	dermatitis
dextr/o	right	dextroscoliosis

I. FILL IN THE BLANK.
Enter the words in the space provided.

1. plasmacytoma_____

2. hexadactylism_____

3. dental_____

4. dermatitis_____

5. dextroscoliosis_____

II. MATCHING.
Match the appropriate terms below.

1. ____ dent/o

2. ____ dextr/o

3. ____ dermat/o

4. ____ cyt/o

5. ____ dactyl/o

A. skin
B. finger/toe
C. cell
D. teeth
E. right

III. MULTIPLE CHOICE.
Choose the appropriate answer for each.

1. Dextr/o deals with the (◯right, ◯ left) side.

2. Dental deals with the (◯teeth, ◯ nails).

3. Dactyl/o deals with the (◯finger/toe, ◯ nails/hair).

4. Cyt/o means (◯nucleus, ◯ cell).

5. Dermat/o means (◯skin, ◯ organs).

Review: Lessons 9–12

I. MATCHING.
Match the appropriate terms below. Some terms may be used more than once.

1. ____ cutane/o		A. fetal covering
2. ____ dent/o		B. finger/toe
3. ____ crypt/o		C. skin
4. ____ cholecyst/o		D. colon
5. ____ cyan/o		E. right
6. ____ dactyl/o		F. cold
7. ____ chol/e		G. teeth
8. ____ dermat/o		H. cartilage
9. ____ cyt/o		I. coccyx
10. ____ colp/o		J. cell
11. ____ dextr/o		K. rib
12. ____ crani/o		L. clavicle
13. ____ chori/o		M. cranium/skull
14. ____ cyst/o		N. bile
15. ____ cry/o		O. blue
16. ____ clavicul/o		P. gallbladder
17. ____ col/o		Q. bladder
18. ____ cost/o		R. conceal
19. ____ chondr/o		S. vagina
20. ____ coccyg/o		

II. TRUE/FALSE.
Determine if the following statements are true or false.

1. You would know the gallbladder is involved if you saw the combining form of cholecyst/o.

   ○ true
   ○ false

2. Hexa- means six. The condition of having six fingers would be hexadactole.

   ○ true
   ○ false

3. A combining form which means skin is durmat/o.
   ○ true
   ○ false

4. Craniocervic/o would indicate the junction between the cranium and neck.
   ○ true
   ○ false

5. Cold is indicated by the combining form criy/o.
   ○ true
   ○ false

6. The correct spelling of the combining form for the area between the rib and the cartilage is costochondr/o.
   ○ true
   ○ false

7. The suffix -rrhaphy means suture. Therefore suturing of the vagina would involve using the combining form of chole/o.
   ○ true
   ○ false

8. To indicate a condition of the skin, a likely combining form would be skin/o.
   ○ true
   ○ false

9. If something is hidden, a likely combining form would be crypt/o.
   ○ true
   ○ false

10. Coal/o means bile.
    ○ true
    ○ false

Root Words – Lesson 13 (Di–Du)

Following is a list of combining forms with their accompanying meanings and a sample word. Memorize these combining forms for the subsequent exercises.

Word Part	Meaning	Example
dips/o	thirst	polydipsia
disc/o	disc/disk	discogenic
dist/o	far/distant from origin	distally

| dors/o | directed toward/on the back | dorsal |
| duoden/o | duodenum | duodenal |

I. FILL IN THE BLANK.
Enter the words in the space provided.

1. polydipsia _____

2. discogenic _____

3. distally _____

4. dorsal _____

5. duodenal _____

II. MATCHING.
Match the appropriate terms below.

1. ____ dips/o

2. ____ disc/o

3. ____ dist/o

4. ____ dors/o

5. ____ duoden/o

A. directed toward/on the back

B. disc

C. thirst

D. distant from origin

E. duodenum

III. MISSING LETTERS.
In the following exercises there are letters missing from each term. Enter the completed term in the space provided.

1. _olyd_psia _____

2. d__sal _____

3. dis_oge_ic _____

4. duo_ena_ _____

5. distal__ _____

Root Words – Lesson 14 (Ec–Er)

Following is a list of combining forms with their accompanying meanings and a sample word. Memorize these combining forms for the subsequent exercises.

Word Part	Meaning	Example
ech/o	sound	echogram
electr/o	electricity	electrodermal
encephal/o	brain	encephalomalacia

| enter/o | intestine | enterocolitis |
| erythr/o | red | erythrocyte |

I. FILL IN THE BLANK.
Enter the words in the space provided.

1. echogram _____

2. electrodermal _____

3. encephalomalacia _____

4. enterocolitis _____

5. erythrocyte _____

II. MATCHING.
Match the appropriate terms below.

1. ____ encephal/o

2. ____ ech/o

3. ____ erythr/o

4. ____ electr/o

5. ____ enter/o

A. red
B. sound
C. brain
D. intestine
E. electricity

III. SPELLING.
Determine if the following words are spelled correctly. If the spelling is correct, leave the word as it has already been entered. If this spelling is incorrect, enter the word with the correct spelling.

1. interocolitis _____

2. electrodermal _____

3. encefalomalacia _____

4. erithrocite _____

5. echogram _____

Root Words – Lesson 15 (Es–Fi)

Following is a list of combining forms with their accompanying meanings and a sample word. Memorize these combining forms for the subsequent exercises.

Word Part	Meaning	Example
esophag/o	esophagus	esophageal
esthesi/o	feeling	anesthesia
femor/o	femur	femoral

fet/o	fetus	fetal
fibr/o	fiber	fibroma

I. FILL IN THE BLANK.
Enter the words in the space provided.

1. esophageal _____

2. anesthesia _____

3. femoral _____

4. fetal _____

5. fibroma _____

II. MATCHING.
Match the appropriate terms below.

1. ____ esophag/o

2. ____ fibr/o

3. ____ esthesi/o

4. ____ fet/o

5. ____ femor/o

A. fetus

B. femur

C. esophagus

D. feeling

E. fiber

III. TRUE/FALSE.
Determine if the following statements are true or false. You need not be concerned with any suffixes you have not been exposed to at this point, as they will be presented in a future lesson.

1. The combining form esophag/o deals with the esophagus.

   ○ true
   ○ false

2. Fetal means fine.

   ○ true
   ○ false

3. The combining form for fiber is fibri/o.

   ○ true
   ○ false

4. The combining form esthesi/o means touching.

○ true
○ false

5. Femoral indicates the femur.

○ true
○ false

Root Words – Lesson 16 (Fi–Ge)

Following is a list of combining forms with their accompanying meanings and a sample word. Memorize these combining forms for the subsequent exercises.

Word Part	Meaning	Example
fibul/o	fibula	fibulotibial
front/o	forehead/front	frontalis
galact/o	milk	galactorrhea
gastr/o	stomach	gastrectomy
genit/o	genitals	genitourinary

I. FILL IN THE BLANK.
Enter the words in the space provided.

1. fibulotibial_____

2. frontalis_____

3. galactorrhea_____

4. gastrectomy_____

5. genitourinary_____

II. MATCHING.
Match the appropriate terms below.

1. ____ front/o

2. ____ genit/o

3. ____ fibul/o

4. ____ gastr/o

5. ____ galact/o

A. stomach
B. milk
C. forehead
D. fibula
E. genitals

III. MULTIPLE CHOICE.
Choose the appropriate answer for each.

1. Gastr/o is the combining form for the (◯ cranium, ◯ stomach).

2. Front/o refers to the (◯ back, ◯ front).

3. Genit/o means (◯ genuine, ◯ genitals).

4. Fibul/o refers to (◯ fiber, ◯ fibula).

5. Galact/o refers to (◯ galaxy, ◯ milk).

Review: Lessons 13–16

I. MATCHING.
Match the appropriate terms below.

1. ____ duoden/o
2. ____ disc/o
3. ____ fibr/o
4. ____ encephal/o
5. ____ galact/o
6. ____ gastr/o
7. ____ ech/o
8. ____ genit/o
9. ____ erythr/o
10. ____ fet/o
11. ____ dist/o
12. ____ dips/o
13. ____ electr/o
14. ____ front/o
15. ____ dors/o
16. ____ fibul/o
17. ____ femor/o
18. ____ enter/o
19. ____ esthesi/o
20. ____ esophag/o

A. forehead
B. femur
C. far
D. thirst
E. brain
F. intestine
G. milk
H. sound
I. stomach
J. electricity
K. fibula
L. esophagus
M. fetus
N. fiber
O. red
P. genitals
Q. disc
R. directed toward/on the back
S. duodenum
T. feeling

II. TRUE/FALSE.
The following words are spelled correctly: true or false?

1. esofageal

○ true
○ false

2. femoral

○ true
○ false

3. frontalis

○ true
○ false

4. polidypsia

○ true
○ false

5. echogram

○ true
○ false

6. fibulotibeal

○ true
○ false

7. duodenal

○ true
○ false

8. electidermal

○ true
○ false

9. gastrectomy

○ true
○ false

10. erythrocyte

○ true
○ false

Root Words – Lesson 17 (Ge–Gn)

Following is a list of combining forms with their accompanying meanings and a sample word. Memorize these combining forms for the subsequent exercises.

Word Part	Meaning	Example
ger/o	old	geriatric
glomerul/o	glomerulus	glomerulonephritis
gloss/o	tongue	glossotonsillar

| glyc/o | sugar/sweet | hyperglycemia |
| gnath/o | jaw | gnathodynia |

I. FILL IN THE BLANK.
Enter the words in the space provided.

1. geriatrics _____

2. glomerulonephritis _____

3. glossotonsillar _____

4. hyperglycemia _____

5. gnathodynia _____

II. MATCHING.
Match the appropriate terms below.

1. ____ gloss/o

2. ____ ger/o

3. ____ gnath/o

4. ____ glomerul/o

5. ____ glyc/o

A. jaw
B. glomerulus
C. old
D. tongue
E. sugar

III. MISSING LETTERS.
In the following exercises there are letters missing from each term. Enter the completed term in the space provided.

1. glos_otonsi__ar _____

2. g_ria_ric _____

3. h_pergl_cem_a _____

4. _nat_odynia _____

5. glom_rulo_ephri_is _____

Root Words – Lesson 18 (Gr–Hi)

Following is a list of combining forms with their accompanying meanings and a sample word. Memorize these combining forms for the subsequent exercises.

Word Part	Meaning	Example
granul/o	grain/particle	granulocyte
gynec/o	female	gynecology

hem/a hem/o hemat/o	blood	hematochezia
hepat/o	liver	hepatomegaly
hist/o	tissue	histoplasmosis

I. **FILL IN THE BLANK.**
Enter the words in the space provided.

1. granulocyte_____

2. gynecology_____

3. hematochezia_____

4. hepatomegaly_____

5. histoplasmosis_____

II. **MATCHING.**
Match the appropriate terms below.

1. ____ gynec/o

2. ____ hepat/o

3. ____ hist/o

4. ____ granul/o

5. ____ hemat/o

A. grain
B. blood
C. female
D. liver
E. tissue

III. **TRUE/FALSE.**
Mark the following true or false.

1. Gynec/o means female.
   ○ true
   ○ false

2. Hepat/o means stomach.
   ○ true
   ○ false

3. The word part for tissue is hyst/o.
   ○ true
   ○ false

4. Both hemat/o and hem/o mean blood.

   ⭕ true
   ⭕ false

5. Granul/o means grain or particle.

   ⭕ true
   ⭕ false

Root Words – Lesson 19 (Ho–II)

Following is a list of combining forms with their accompanying meanings and a sample word. Memorize these combining forms for the subsequent exercises.

Word Part	Meaning	Example
hom/o	common/same	homogeneous
humer/o	humerus	humeral
hydr/o	water	hydrometer
hyster/o	uterus/womb	hysterosalpingogram
ile/o	ileum (small intestine)	ileocecal

I. **FILL IN THE BLANK.**
   Enter the words in the space provided.

1. homogeneous _____

2. humeral _____

3. hydrometer _____

4. hysterosalpingogram _____

5. ileocecal _____

II. MATCHING.
Match the appropriate terms below.

1. ____ hydr/o
2. ____ hyster/o
3. ____ ile/o
4. ____ hom/o
5. ____ humer/o

A. common/same
B. water
C. humerus
D. ileum
E. uterus

III. UNSCRAMBLE.
Unscramble each of the following words based on information presented in this unit. Enter the complete word in the blank provided.

1. esmooounehg _____

2. romdetrehy _____

3. remaluh _____

4. alceoelci _____

5. rosmargogytsehalpni _____

Root Words – Lesson 20 (Il–Ir)

Following is a list of combining forms with their accompanying meanings and a sample word. Memorize these combining forms for the subsequent exercises.

Word Part	Meaning	Example
ili/o	ilium (hip bone)	sacroiliac
immun/o	immune	immunodeficiency
infer/o	lowermost/below	inferior
intestin/o	intestine	gastrointestinal
irid/o	colored circle/iris	iridectomy

I. FILL IN THE BLANK.
Enter the words in the space provided.

1. sacroiliac_____

2. immunodeficiency_____

3. inferior_____

4. gastrointestinal_____

5. iridectomy_____

II. MATCHING.
Match the appropriate terms below.

1. ____ ili/o

2. ____ irid/o

3. ____ intestin/o

4. ____ infer/o

5. ____ immun/o

A. immune

B. lowermost/below

C. ilium

D. intestine

E. colored circle

III. MULTIPLE CHOICE.
Choose the correct answer.

1. The root word for lowermost is (◯unfer/o, ◯ infer/o).

2. Irid/o means (◯pupil, ◯ iris).

3. The combining form for immune is (◯immun/o, ◯ immune/o).

4. The combining for intestine is (◯intesine/o, ◯ intestin/o).

Review: Lessons 17–20

I. MATCHING.
Match the appropriate terms below.

1. ____ ili/o
2. ____ hom/o
3. ____ immun/o
4. ____ hist/o
5. ____ ile/o
6. ____ intestin/o
7. ____ hepat/o
8. ____ humer/o
9. ____ hyster/o
10. ____ gloss/o
11. ____ hydr/o
12. ____ infer/o
13. ____ gnath/o
14. ____ irid/o
15. ____ gynec/o
16. ____ glomerul/ o
17. ____ glyc/o
18. ____ ger/o
19. ____ granul/o
20. ____ hem/o

A. old
B. colored circle
C. sugar
D. lowermost/below
E. small intestine
F. grain
G. female
H. immune
I. liver
J. blood
K. jaw
L. glomerulus
M. uterus
N. tongue
O. water
P. tissue
Q. same
R. humerus
S. hip bone
T. intestine

II. SPELLING.
Determine if the following words are spelled correctly. If the spelling is correct, leave the word as it has already been entered. If this spelling is incorrect, enter the word with the correct spelling.

1. himogenous _____
2. infiror _____
3. sacroileac _____
4. iridectomy _____
5. hidrometer _____
6. geriatric _____

7. gynecology _____   8. gnathodynia _____

9. glomerolus _____   10. hepatimegaly _____

Root Words – Lesson 21 (Is–La)

Following is a list of combining forms with their accompanying meanings and a sample word. Memorize these combining forms for the subsequent exercises.

Word Part	Meaning	Example
ischi/o	ischium	ischiodynia
jejun/o	jejunum	jejunostomy
labi/o	lip	labial
lacrim/o	tear/crying	lacrimal
lact/o	milk	lactose

I. FILL IN THE BLANK.
Enter the words in the space provided.

1. ischiodynia _____   2. jejunostomy _____

3. labial _____   4. lacrimal _____

5. lactose _____

II. MATCHING.
Match the appropriate terms below.

1. ____ lact/o

2. ____ lacrim/o

3. ____ labi/o

4. ____ ischi/o

5. ____ jejun/o

A. ischium
B. lip
C. jejunum
D. tear/crying
E. milk

III. FILL IN THE BLANK.
Enter the appropriate term in the space provided using the terms in this lesson.

1. The combining form labi/o means _____.

2. The combining form for the word ischium is _____.

3. Lact/o means _____.

4. The combining form for crying is _____.

5. Jejun/o is the combining form for _____.

Root Words – Lesson 22 (La–Li)

Following is a list of combining forms with their accompanying meanings and a sample word. Memorize these combining forms for the subsequent exercises.

Word Part	Meaning	Example
lapar/o	flank/abdominal wall	laparoscope
laryng/o	larynx (voice box)	laryngeal
later/o	side	anterolateral
leuc/o leuk/o	white	leukocyte
lingu/o	tongue	lingula

I. FILL IN THE BLANK.
Enter the words in the space provided.

1. laparoscope _____

2. laryngeal _____

3. anterolateral _____

4. leukocyte _____

5. lingula _____

II. MATCHING.
Match the appropriate terms below.

1. ___ lapar/o
2. ___ later/o
3. ___ laryng/o
4. ___ leuk/o
5. ___ lingu/o

A. tongue
B. side
C. white
D. flank
E. larynx

III. MISSING LETTERS.
In the following exercises there are letters missing from each term. Enter the completed term in the space provided.

1. l_uk_cyte _____

2. _ingu_a _____

3. laryn_ _ al _____

4. l_parosc_pe _____

5. anter_lat_ral _____

Root Words – Lesson 23 (Li–Ly)

Following is a list of combining forms with their accompanying meanings and a sample word. Memorize these combining forms for the subsequent exercises.

Word Part	Meaning	Example
lip/o	fat	liposuction
lith/o	stone	cholelithiasis
lob/o	lobe	lobular
lumb/o	lower back	lumbosacral
lymph/o	lymph/lymphatics	lymph nodes

I. FILL IN THE BLANK.
Enter the words in the space provided.

1. liposuction _____

2. cholelithiasis _____

3. lobular _____

4. lumbosacral _____

5. lymph nodes _____

II. MATCHING.
Match the appropriate terms below.

1. ____ lith/o
2. ____ lip/o
3. ____ lymph/o
4. ____ lumb/o
5. ____ lob/o

A. lower back
B. lymph
C. fat
D. stone
E. lobe

III. MULTIPLE CHOICE.
Choose the best answer.

1. Lith/o means (◯ stone, ◯ black).

2. The lower back would be indicated by (◯ lumbi/o, ◯ lumb/o).

3. Lob/o means (◯ low, ◯ lobe).

4. Lymph/o means (◯ lymph node(s), ◯ lactose).

5. Lip/o indicates (◯ fat, ◯ lips).

Root Words – Lesson 24 (Ma–Me)

Following is a list of combining forms with their accompanying meanings and a sample word. Memorize these combining forms for the subsequent exercises.

Word Part	Meaning	Example
mamm/o mast/o	breast	mammogram/mastectomy
medi/o	middle	mediolateral
melan/o	black	melanotic
men/o	month	dysmenorrhea
mening/o	membrane	meningocele

I. FILL IN THE BLANK.
Enter the words in the space provided.

1. mammogram _____

2. mastectomy _____

3. mediolateral _____

4. melanotic _____

5. dysmenorrhea _____

6. meningocele _____

II. MATCHING.
Match the appropriate terms below.

1. ____ men/o

2. ____ mening/o

3. ____ mast/o

4. ____ medi/o

5. ____ melan/o

A. breast
B. black
C. month
D. membrane
E. middle

III. UNSCRAMBLE.
Unscramble each of the following words based on information presented in this unit. Enter the complete word in the blank provided.

1. alraetioldem _____

2. geninmoceel _____

3. cimenalto _____

4. magrommam _____

5. ymotcetsam _____

Review: Lessons 21–24

I. MATCHING.
Match the appropriate terms below.

1. ____ laryng/o
2. ____ ischi/o
3. ____ later/o
4. ____ men/o
5. ____ labi/o
6. ____ mamm/o
7. ____ lact/o
8. ____ lapar/o
9. ____ lymph/o
10. ____ jejun/o
11. ____ leuk/o
12. ____ lumb/o
13. ____ mening/o
14. ____ lacrim/o
15. ____ medi/o
16. ____ lip/o
17. ____ lob/o
18. ____ lith/o
19. ____ lingu/o
20. ____ melan/o

A. stone
B. tongue
C. jejunum
D. tear/crying
E. flank
F. white
G. lower back
H. ischium
I. milk
J. membrane
K. lobe
L. middle
M. side
N. lymph
O. black
P. larynx
Q. breast
R. month
S. lip
T. fat

II. TRUE/FALSE.
Mark the following true or false.

1. The combining form men/o means men/male.

   ○ true
   ○ false

2. Medi/o refers to the middle.

   ○ true
   ○ false

3. The combining form for tongue is tong/o.
   ○ true
   ○ false

4. Both leuc/o and leuk/o are acceptable combining forms for the word white.
   ○ true
   ○ false

5. The ischium is the hip.
   ○ true
   ○ false

6. The combining form for stone is leth/o.
   ○ true
   ○ false

7. Mening/o means mouth.
   ○ true
   ○ false

8. The larynx is the voice box.
   ○ true
   ○ false

9. Black is represented by the combining form of melan/o.
   ○ true
   ○ false

10. The abdominal wall is also the flank.
    ○ true
    ○ false

Root Words – Lesson 25 (Me–My)

Following is a list of combining forms with their accompanying meanings and a sample word. Memorize these combining forms for the subsequent exercises.

Word Part	Meaning	Example
metr/i	uterine tissue	endometritis
mon/o	one/only	monoclonal
muc/o	mucus	mucoperiosteal

| muscul/o | muscle | musculotendinous |
| my/o | muscle | myometrium |

I. FILL IN THE BLANK.
Enter the words in the space provided.

1. endometritis _____

2. monoclonal _____

3. mucoperiosteal _____

4. musculotendinous _____

5. myometrium _____

II. MATCHING.
Match the appropriate terms below.

1. ____ muscul/o

2. ____ metr/i

3. ____ mon/o

4. ____ my/o

5. ____ muc/o

A. one
B. mucus
C. muscle
D. uterine tissue

III. MISSING LETTERS.
In the following exercises there are letters missing from each term. Enter the completed term in the space provided.

1. muc_periost_al _____

2. _on_clona_ _____

3. endom_trit_s _____

4. m_ome_ri_m _____

5. muscul_ten_inou_ _____

Root Words – Lesson 26 (My–Ne)

Following is a list of combining forms with their accompanying meanings and a sample word. Memorize these combining forms for the subsequent exercises.

Word Part	Meaning	Example
myc/o	fungus	mycosis
myel/o	marrow/spinal cord	myeloma

narc/o	sleep/numbness	narcolepsy
nas/o	nose	nasopharyngeal
ne/o	new	neoblastic

I. FILL IN THE BLANK.
Enter the words in the space provided.

1. mycosis _____

2. myeloma _____

3. narcolepsy _____

4. nasopharyngeal _____

5. neoblastic _____

II. MATCHING.
Match the appropriate terms below.

1. ____ myel/o

2. ____ myc/o

3. ____ narc/o

4. ____ nas/o

5. ____ ne/o

A. nose
B. new
C. marrow
D. fungus
E. sleep

III. TRUE/FALSE.
Determine if the following statements are true or false.

1. Narc/o means awake.
   ○ true
   ○ false

2. Myc/o indicates muscle.
   ○ true
   ○ false

3. Nas/o is the combining form for nose.
   ○ true
   ○ false

4. Ne/o is the combining form for new.

○ true
○ false

5. Myel/o means marrow or spinal cord.

○ true
○ false

Root Words – Lesson 27 (Ne–Od)

Following is a list of combining forms with their accompanying meanings and a sample word. Memorize these combining forms for the subsequent exercises.

Word Part	Meaning	Example
necr/o	dead/corpse	necrosis
nephr/o	kidney	nephrolithiasis
neur/o	nerves	neuritis
odont/o	teeth	odontoid
odyn/o	pain/distress	odynophagia

I. **FILL IN THE BLANK.**
   Enter the words in the space provided.

   1. necrosis _____

   2. nephrolithiasis _____

   3. neuritis _____

   4. odontoid _____

   5. odynophagia _____

II. **MATCHING.**
   Match the appropriate terms below.

   1. ____ nephr/o

   2. ____ odont/o

   3. ____ odyn/o

   4. ____ neur/o

   5. ____ necr/o

   A. nerve
   B. dead
   C. kidney
   D. teeth
   E. pain

III. FILL IN THE BLANK.
Enter the appropriate term in the space provided using the terms in this lesson.

1. Nephr/o is the combining form for _____.

2. Pain or distress is indicated by the combining form of _____.

3. Odont/o is the combining form for _____.

4. _____ is the combining form for nerves.

5. Death is indicated by the combining form of _____.

Root Words – Lesson 28 (On–Or)

Following is a list of combining forms with their accompanying meanings and a sample word. Memorize these combining forms for the subsequent exercises.

Word Part	Meaning	Example
onc/o	bulk/tumor	oncology
oophor/o	ovary	oophorosalpingitis
ophthalm/o	eye	ophthalmology
or/o	mouth	intraoral
orchi/o	testicle	orchiectomy

I. FILL IN THE BLANK.
Enter the words in the space provided.

1. oncology _____

2. oophorosalpingitis _____

3. ophthalmology _____

4. intraoral _____

5. orchiectomy _____

II. MATCHING.
Match the appropriate terms below.

1. ____ orchi/o
2. ____ oophor/o
3. ____ onc/o
4. ____ or/o
5. ____ ophthalm/o

A. ovary
B. mouth
C. eye
D. testicle
E. tumor

III. UNSCRAMBLE.
Unscramble each of the following words based on information presented in this unit. Enter the complete word in the blank provided.

1. ygolonco _____

2. laroarnit _____

3. oygolmalhhtpo _____

4. ceitoymhocr _____

5. siitgpinlasooroohp _____

Review: Lessons 25–28

I. MATCHING.
Match the appropriate terms below.

1. ____ or/o
2. ____ ne/o
3. ____ myel/o
4. ____ onc/o
5. ____ orchi/o
6. ____ narc/o
7. ____ metr/i
8. ____ mon/o
9. ____ nas/o
10. ____ neur/o
11. ____ ophthalm/o
12. ____ odont/o
13. ____ oophor/o
14. ____ odyn/o
15. ____ nephr/o
16. ____ muc/o
17. ____ necr/o
18. ____ muscul/o
19. ____ my/o
20. ____ myc/o

A. only
B. marrow/spinal cord
C. ovary
D. uterine tissue
E. sleep
F. mucus
G. tumor
H. testicle
I. mouth
J. teeth
K. dead
L. new
M. eye
N. nose
O. nerve
P. pain
Q. kidney
R. fungus
S. muscle

II. MULTIPLE CHOICE.
Choose the correct answer.

1. The combining form for nerves is (◯ner/o,◯ neur/o).

2. (◯Ne/o,◯ New/o) means new.

3. The correct combining form for sleep is (◯sleep/o,◯ narc/o).

4. Mouth is indicated by (◯orou/o,◯ or/o).

5. Testicle is indicated by (◯test/o,◯ orchi/o).

6. (◯Oophor/o,◯ Ophthalm/o) means eye.

7. To indicate one, the combining form (◯mon/o,◯ one/o) would be used.

8. (◯My/o,◯ Myc/o) means muscle.

9. Uterine tissue is indicated by the combining form of (◯colp/o,◯ metr/i).

10. Muscul/o and my/o both mean (◯much,◯ muscle).

Root Words – Lesson 29 (Or–Pa)

Following is a list of combining forms with their accompanying meanings and a sample word. Memorize these combining forms for the subsequent exercises.

Word Part	Meaning	Example
orth/o	straight	orthopedic
oste/o	bone	osteopathic
ot/o	ear	otolaryngology
pancreat/o	pancreas	pancreatitis
patell/o	patella (kneecap)	patellofemoral

I. **FILL IN THE BLANK.**
   Enter the words in the space provided.

1. orthopedic_____

2. osteopathic_____

3. otolaryngology_____

4. pancreatitis_____

5. patellofemoral_____

II. MATCHING.
Match the appropriate terms below.

1. ____ orth/o
2. ____ patell/o
3. ____ ot/o
4. ____ oste/o
5. ____ pancreat/o

A. ear
B. bone
C. pancreas
D. straight
E. kneecap

III. TRUE/FALSE.
Determine if the following statements are true or false. You need not be concerned with any suffixes you have not been exposed to at this point, as they will be presented in a future lesson.

1. Patellofemoral involves the elbow.
   ○ true
   ○ false

2. Oste/o means straight.
   ○ true
   ○ false

3. Ear is represented by the combining form of ear/o.
   ○ true
   ○ false

4. The pancreas is represented by the combining form of pancreat/o.
   ○ true
   ○ false

5. Orth/o means straight.
   ○ true
   ○ false

Root Words – Lesson 30 (Pa–Ph)

Following is a list of combining forms with their accompanying meanings and a sample word. Memorize these combining forms for the subsequent exercises.

Word Part	Meaning	Example
path/o	disease	pathologist
pelv/i	pelvis	pelvimetry

periton/o	peritoneum	intraperitoneal
pharmac/o	drugs/medicine	pharmacological
pharyng/o	pharynx	cricopharyngeal

I. FILL IN THE BLANK.
Enter the words in the space provided.

1. pathologist_____

2. pelvimetry_____

3. intraperitoneal_____

4. pharmacological_____

5. cricopharyngeal_____

II. MATCHING.
Match the appropriate terms below.

1. ____ pelv/i

2. ____ pharyng/o

3. ____ periton/o

4. ____ path/o

5. ____ pharmac/o

A. disease
B. drugs
C. pharynx
D. peritoneum
E. pelvis

III. SPELLING.
Determine if the following words are spelled correctly. If the spelling is correct, leave the word as it has been entered. If this spelling is incorrect, enter the word with the correct spelling.

1. interperitoneal _____

2. pathologist _____

3. pelvemetry _____

4. cricofaryngeal _____

5. pharmacologecal _____

Root Words – Lesson 31 (Ph–Pl)

Following is a list of combining forms with their accompanying meanings and a sample word. Memorize these combining forms for the subsequent exercises.

Word Part	Meaning	Example
phleb/o	vein	phlebolith
phon/o	sound/voice	phonation
phot/o	light	photophobia

| phren/o | mind/diaphragm | costophrenic |
| pleur/o | pleura | pleurodesis |

I. FILL IN THE BLANK.
Enter the words in the space provided.

1. phlebolith _____

2. phonation _____

3. photophobia _____

4. costophrenic _____

5. pleurodesis _____

II. MATCHING.
Match the appropriate terms below.

1. ____ phot/o

2. ____ pleur/o

3. ____ phleb/o

4. ____ phren/o

5. ____ phon/o

A. vein
B. sound
C. diaphragm
D. pleura
E. light

III. UNSCRAMBLE.
Unscramble each of the following words based on information presented in this unit. Enter the complete word in the blank provided.

1. anohpniot _____

2. crctoosinehp _____

3. sidesorulep _____

4. paibohpooht _____

5. htilbolphe _____

Root Words – Lesson 32 (Po–Pr)

Following is a list of combining forms with their accompanying meanings and a sample word. Memorize these combining forms for the subsequent exercises.

Word Part	Meaning	Example
poster/o	posterior/toward back	posterolateral
pneum/o	air/breathing/lung	pneumothorax
proct/o	rectum/anus	proctitis

prostat/o	prostate	prostatectomy
proxim/o	nearest point of origin	proximal

I. FILL IN THE BLANK.
Enter the words in the space provided.

1. posterolateral _____

2. pneumothorax _____

3. proctitis _____

4. prostatectomy _____

5. proximal _____

II. MATCHING.
Match the appropriate terms below.

1. ____ pneum/o

2. ____ proxim/o

3. ____ poster/o

4. ____ prostat/o

5. ____ proct/o

A. prostate
B. breathing
C. anus
D. toward the back
E. nearest to the point of origin

III. MISSING LETTERS.
In the following exercises there are letters missing from each term. Enter the completed term in the space provided.

1. pr_ximal _____

2. _ _octitis _____

3. pr_sta_ecto_y _____

4. pne_ _othora_ _____

5. post_rolater_l _____

Review: Lessons 29–32

I. MATCHING.
Match the appropriate terms below.

1. ___ ot/o		A.	air/breathing
2. ___ prostat/o		B.	pharynx
3. ___ oste/o		C.	rectum
4. ___ pneum/o		D.	ear
5. ___ proct/o		E.	bone
6. ___ pelv/i		F.	nearest point of origin
7. ___ proxim/o		G.	kneecap
8. ___ periton/o		H.	disease
9. ___ orth/o		I.	drugs
10. ___ pharyng/o		J.	pelvis
11. ___ path/o		K.	prostate
12. ___ patell/o		L.	pancreas
13. ___ poster/o		M.	straight
14. ___ phleb/o		N.	peritoneum
15. ___ pleur/o		O.	pleura
16. ___ phot/o		P.	vein
17. ___ phren/o		Q.	sound
18. ___ phon/o		R.	light
19. ___ pancreat/o		S.	toward the back
20. ___ pharmac/o		T.	diaphragm

II. MULTIPLE CHOICE.
Choose the correct answer.

1. The combining form which means lung or breathing is (◯ lung/o, ◯ pneum/o).

2. Phot/o means (◯ dark, ◯ light).

3. Phren/o indicates both mind and (◯ diaphragm, ◯ vision).

4. The rectum is indicated by the combining form of (◯ proct/o, ◯ prostat/o).

5. Phon/o means (◯ phony, ◯ sound).

6. The combining form for vein is (◯ phleb/o, ◯ fleb/o).

7. Path/o means (◯ disease, ◯ path).

8. The pelvis is indicated by the combining form (◯ pelv/i, ◯ pilv/o).

9. The combining form for bone is (◯ osti/o, ◯ oste/o).

10. Another name for the patella is the (◯ elbow, ◯ kneecap).

Root Words – Lesson 33 (Ps–Py)

Following is a list of combining forms with their accompanying meanings and a sample word. Memorize these combining forms for the subsequent exercises.

Word Part	Meaning	Example
pseud/o	false	pseudarthrosis
psych/o	mind	psychiatry
pub/o	pubis	pubococcygeal
pulm/o pulmon/o	lung	pulmonary
py/o	pus	pyoid

I. **FILL IN THE BLANK.**
   Enter the words in the space provided.

1. pseudarthrosis_____   2. psychiatry_____

3. pubococcygeal_____   4. pulmonary_____

5. pyoid_____

II. MATCHING.
Match the appropriate terms below.

1. ____ py/o
2. ____ psych/o
3. ____ pub/o
4. ____ pseud/o
5. ____ pulm/o

A. false
B. lung
C. mind
D. pus
E. pubis

III. TRUE/FALSE.
The following words are spelled correctly: true or false?

1. pulminary
   ○ true
   ○ false

2. pioid
   ○ true
   ○ false

3. psuedoarthrosis
   ○ true
   ○ false

4. pubococcygeal
   ○ true
   ○ false

5. psychiatry
   ○ true
   ○ false

Root Words – Lesson 34 (Py–Rh)

Following is a list of combining forms with their accompanying meanings and a sample word. Memorize these combining forms for the subsequent exercises.

Word Part	Meaning	Example
pyel/o	trough/renal pelvis	pyelogram
radi/o	radius/radiant energy	radiology
rect/o	rectum	rectal

| ren/o | kidneys | renal |
| rhin/o | nose | rhinoplasty |

I. FILL IN THE BLANK.
Enter the words in the space provided.

1. pyelogram_____

2. radiology_____

3. rectal_____

4. renal_____

5. rhinoplasty_____

II. MATCHING.
Match the appropriate terms below.

1. ____ ren/o

2. ____ pyel/o

3. ____ rhin/o

4. ____ rect/o

5. ____ radi/o

A. nose
B. rectum
C. radiant energy/radius
D. kidneys
E. trough/renal pelvis

III. FILL IN THE BLANK.
Enter the appropriate term in the space provided using the terms in this lesson.

1. The correct combining form for kidneys is _____.

2. To indicate nose, one would use the combining form of _____.

3. Rect/o as a combining form means _____.

4. _____ is the combining form for renal pelvis.

5. _____ is the combining form for radiant energy.

Root Words – Lesson 35 (Sa–Se)

Following is a list of combining forms with their accompanying meanings and a sample word. Memorize these combining forms for the subsequent exercises.

Word Part	Meaning	Example
sacr/o	sacrum	lumbosacral
salping/o	tube	salpingo-oophorectomy

scrot/o	scrotum	scrotal
semin/o	semen	seminal
ser/o	serum	serosanguineous

I. FILL IN THE BLANK.
Enter the words in the space provided.

1. lumbosacral _____

2. salpingo-oophorectomy _____

3. scrotal _____

4. seminal _____

5. serosanguineous _____

II. MATCHING.
Match the appropriate terms below.

1. ____ sacr/o

2. ____ scrot/o

3. ____ semin/o

4. ____ ser/o

5. ____ salping/o

A. scrotum
B. tube
C. sacrum
D. semen
E. serum

III. TRUE/FALSE.
Mark the following true or false.

1. Ser/o means circle.
   ○ true
   ○ false

2. Salping/o means tube.
   ○ true
   ○ false

3. Scrotum is indicated by the combining form of scrot/o.
   ○ true
   ○ false

4. Semin/o means semen.

   ○ true
   ○ false

5. Sacr/o means scared.

   ○ true
   ○ false

Root Words – Lesson 36 (So–Sp)

Following is a list of combining forms with their accompanying meanings and a sample word. Memorize these combining forms for the subsequent exercises.

Word Part	Meaning	Example
somat/o	body	somatization
son/o	sound	sonogram
spermat/o	seed	spermatocele
sphen/o	wedge/sphenoid	sphenoethmoid
splen/o	spleen	hepatosplenomegaly

I. FILL IN THE BLANK.
Enter the words in the space provided.

1. somatization_____

2. sonogram_____

3. spermatocele_____

4. sphenoethmoid_____

5. hepatosplenomegaly_____

II. MATCHING.
Match the appropriate terms below.

1. ____ sphen/o
2. ____ splen/o
3. ____ somat/o
4. ____ spermat/o
5. ____ son/o

A. body
B. sound
C. wedge
D. spleen
E. seed

III. MISSING LETTERS.
In the following exercises there are letters missing from each term. Enter the completed term in the space provided.

1. s_erma_oce_e _____

2. so_ _tization _____

3. _epatos_lenome_aly _____

4. sp_enoethm_ _ _ _____

5. sono_ram _____

Review: Lessons 33–36

I. MATCHING.
Match the appropriate terms below.

1. ____ rect/o
2. ____ splen/o
3. ____ son/o
4. ____ sacr/o
5. ____ pub/o
6. ____ sphen/o
7. ____ rhin/o
8. ____ psych/o
9. ____ py/o
10. ____ scrot/o
11. ____ spermat/o
12. ____ ren/o
13. ____ pulmon/o
14. ____ pseud/o
15. ____ salping/o
16. ____ somat/o
17. ____ ser/o
18. ____ semin/o
19. ____ pyel/o
20. ____ radi/o

A. false
B. kidneys
C. pus
D. wedge
E. radius
F. mind
G. scrotum
H. spleen
I. nose
J. pubis
K. tube
L. seed
M. renal pelvis
N. sound
O. rectum
P. serum
Q. semen
R. body
S. lung
T. sacrum

II. MULTIPLE CHOICE.
Choose the correct answer.

1. Sphen/o means (◯ wedge, ◯ spleen).

2. A radiologist deals with (◯ radiant energy, ◯ radios).

3. Pyel/o means both renal pelvis and (◯ trough, ◯ pus).

4. Psych/o means (◯ mind, ◯ school).

5. Pulm/o and pulmon/o both mean (◯ pull, ◯ lung).

6. Body is represented by the combining form of (◯ somat/o, ◯ bod/o).

7. Spermat/o means (◯ seed, ◯ sacrum).

8. Pubis is represented by the combining form of (◯ rect/o, ◯ pub/o).

9. Pus is represented by the combining form of (◯ py/o, ◯ pi/o).

Root Words – Lesson 37 (Sp–Te)

Following is a list of combining forms with their accompanying meanings and a sample word. Memorize these combining forms for the subsequent exercises.

Word Part	Meaning	Example
spondyl/o	vertebra	spondylolisthesis
stern/o	sternum	sternocleidomastoid
tars/o	ankle bone (tarsal)	metatarsal
tempor/o	temple	temporomandibular
ten/o	tendon/tight band	tenosynovitis

I. **FILL IN THE BLANK.**
   Enter the words in the space provided.

1. spondylolisthesis _____

2. sternocleidomastoid _____

3. metatarsal _____

4. temporomandibular _____

5. tenosynovitis _____

II. MATCHING.
Match the appropriate terms below.

1. ____ ten/o
2. ____ tempor/o
3. ____ stern/o
4. ____ spondyl/o
5. ____ tars/o

A. vertebra
B. sternum
C. ankle bone
D. temple
E. tendon

III. UNSCRAMBLE.
Unscramble each of the following words based on information presented in this unit. Enter the complete word in the blank provided.

1. lasrtaamet _____
2. raetmpluoomradnbi _____
3. snopyldsieshtsoil _____
4. netstiysoinvo _____
5. ramdtsnocestoiodeil _____

Root Words – Lesson 38 (Th–To)

Following is a list of combining forms with their accompanying meanings and a sample word. Memorize these combining forms for the subsequent exercises.

Word Part	Meaning	Example
therm/o	heat	thermometer
thorac/o	chest	thoracic
thromb/o	clot/thrombus	thrombosis
tibi/o	tibia	tibiotalar
tonsill/o	tonsil	tonsillectomy

I. FILL IN THE BLANK.
Enter the words in the space provided.

1. thermometer _____   2. thoracic _____

3. thrombosis _____   4. tibiotalar _____

5. tonsillectomy _____

II. MATCHING.
Match the appropriate terms below.

1. ____   therm/o

2. ____   tonsill/o

3. ____   thorac/o

4. ____   thromb/o

5. ____   tibi/o

A. chest

B. lump/clot

C. tibia

D. tonsil

E. heat

III. TRUE/FALSE.
The following words are spelled correctly: true or false?

1. thrombosis
   - ○ true
   - ○ false

2. thirmometer
   - ○ true
   - ○ false

3. tonsilectomy
   - ○ true
   - ○ false

4. thoracick
   - ○ true
   - ○ false

5. tibeotalar
   - ○ true
   - ○ false

Root Words – Lesson 39 (To–Ur)

Following is a list of combining forms with their accompanying meanings and a sample word. Memorize these combining forms for the subsequent exercises.

Word Part	Meaning	Example
tox/o	poison	toxemia
trache/o	trachea (windpipe)	tracheotomy
uln/o	ulna	ulnoradial
ur/o	urine	polyuria
ureter/o	ureter	ureterovesical

I. FILL IN THE BLANK.
Enter the words in the space provided.

1. toxemia _____

2. tracheotomy _____

3. ulnoradial _____

4. polyuria _____

5. ureterovesical _____

II. MATCHING.
Match the appropriate terms below.

1. ____ ureter/o

2. ____ uln/o

3. ____ ur/o

4. ____ tox/o

5. ____ trache/o

A. urine
B. windpipe
C. poison
D. ureter
E. ulna

III. FILL IN THE BLANK.
Enter the appropriate term in the space provided using the terms in this lesson.

1. The combining form for urine is _____.

2. Ureter is represented by the combining form of _____.

3. The trachea is also called the _____.

4. _____ is the combining form for ulna.

5. Tox/o is the combining form meaning _____ .

Root Words – Lesson 40 (Ur–Ve)

Following is a list of combining forms with their accompanying meanings and a sample word. Memorize these combining forms for the subsequent exercises.

Word Part	Meaning	Example
urethr/o	urethra	urethritis
uter/o	uterus	uterovaginal
vag/o	vagus nerve	vagotomy
vas/o	vessel/ductus deferens	vasovagal
ven/o	vein	venotomy

I. **FILL IN THE BLANK.**
   Enter the words in the space provided.

1. urethritis _____

2. uterovaginal _____

3. vagotomy _____

4. vasovagal _____

5. venotomy _____

II. **MATCHING.**
   Match the appropriate terms below.

1. ____ urethr/o

2. ____ uter/o

3. ____ vag/o

4. ____ vas/o

5. ____ ven/o

A. vein
B. vessel
C. vagus nerve
D. uterus
E. urethra

III. MISSING LETTERS.
In the following exercises there are letters missing from each term. Enter the completed term in the space provided.

1. ute_ov_ginal _____

2. va_ov_gal _____

3. _rethrit_s _____

4. ven_ _omy _____

5. v_gotomy _____

Root Words – Lesson 41 (Ve–Xa)

Following is a list of combining forms with their accompanying meanings and a sample word. Memorize these combining forms for the subsequent exercises.

Word Part	Meaning	Example
ventr/o	ventral/belly side	ventral
vertebr/o	vertebra	costovertebral
vulv/o	vulva	vulvectomy
xanth/o	yellow	xanthoma

I. FILL IN THE BLANK.
Enter the words in the space provided.

1. ventral _____

2. costovertebral _____

3. vulvectomy _____

4. xanthoma _____

II. MATCHING.
Match the appropriate terms below.

1. ____ vulv/o

2. ____ xanth/o

3. ____ vertebr/o

4. ____ ventr/o

A. vertebra
B. belly side
C. yellow
D. vulva

III. TRUE/FALSE.
The following words are spelled correctly: true or false?

1. chostovertebral

   ○ true
   ○ false

2. ventril

   ○ true
   ○ false

3. zanthoma

   ○ true
   ○ false

4. vulvectomy

   ○ true
   ○ false

5. vulvo

   ○ true
   ○ false

Review: Lessons 37–41

I. **MATCHING.**
   Match the appropriate terms below.

1. ____ ur/o
2. ____ tars/o
3. ____ xanth/o
4. ____ urethr/o
5. ____ stern/o
6. ____ tibi/o
7. ____ ven/o
8. ____ tonsill/o
9. ____ spondyl/o
10. ____ tox/o
11. ____ ventr/o
12. ____ vas/o
13. ____ vulv/o
14. ____ therm/o
15. ____ vag/o
16. ____ ten/o
17. ____ ureter/o
18. ____ tempor/o
19. ____ thromb/o
20. ____ vertebr/o
21. ____ trache/o
22. ____ uln/o
23. ____ thorac/o
24. ____ uter/o

A. heat
B. vein
C. ulna
D. chest
E. urethra
F. temple
G. vertebra
H. vulva
I. clot/thrombus
J. vagus nerve
K. tibia
L. belly side
M. yellow
N. tonsil
O. uterus
P. ankle bone
Q. sternum
R. poison
S. ureter
T. vessel
U. urine
V. tendon
W. trachea

II. MULTIPLE CHOICE.
Choose the correct answer.

1. The combining form for the windpipe is (◯trache/o, ◯track/o).

2. Clot is another word for (◯thrombus, ◯ulna).

3. The tarsal is the (◯ankle bone, ◯kneecap).

4. Tempor/o is the combining form for the word (◯temporary, ◯temple).

5. Tonsill/o indicates (◯tonsill, ◯tonsil).

6. Uln/o is the combining form for (◯ulna, ◯knee).

7. Ductus deferens is also called a (◯vessel, ◯vagina).

8. Xanth/o represents the color (◯black, ◯yellow).

9. Ventr/o means (◯back side, ◯belly side).

10. The combining form for a vein is (◯ven/o, ◯vein/o).

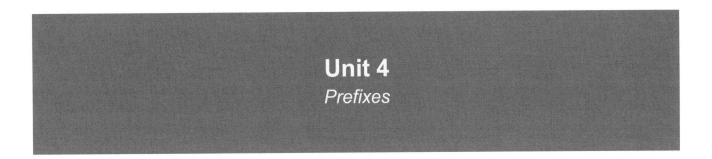

Unit 4
Prefixes

Prefixes – Introduction

A prefix is added to the beginning of a word to modify or change its meaning. With a few exceptions, which will be noted as they occur, prefixes can be added to a word without changing either form, specifically without changing the spelling of the prefix itself or the root word that follows it. Like the root words unit and the suffixes unit (still to come), this unit on prefixes will be presented mostly alphabetically.

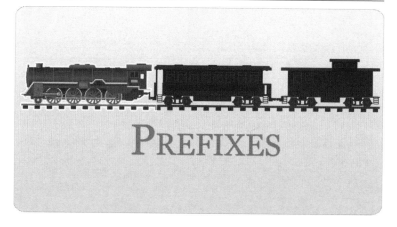

- *Prefixes A–He in Lessons 1–3*
- *Prefixes Hy–Pe in Lessons 4–6*
- *Prefixes Pe–Un in Lesson 7–8*
- *Sound-Alike Prefixes in Lesson 9*
- *Synonymous Prefixes in Lesson 10*

We will begin our study of prefixes with prefixes A–He.

Prefixes – Lesson 1 (A)

Following is a list of prefixes with their accompanying meanings and a sample word. Memorize these prefixes for the subsequent exercises.

Prefix	Meaning	Example
a-/an-	no/without	amenorrhea/anechoic (a- before a consonant, an- before a vowel)
ab-	away from	abduct
ad-	toward	adduct
ante-/pre-/pro-	before	antenatal/preoperative
anti-/contra-	against	antibiotic/contralateral

I. MATCHING.
Match the appropriate terms below.

1. ____ contra-

2. ____ ab-

3. ____ a-

4. ____ ante-

5. ____ ad-

A. without

B. toward

C. before

D. away from

E. against

II. MULTIPLE CHOICE.
Choose the correct answer.

1. The prefix ab- means (◯ without, ◯ toward, ◯ against, ◯ away from).

2. Before birth is (◯ante-, ◯ a-, ◯ad-, ◯contra-) partum.

3. Contralateral means (◯against, ◯toward, ◯before, ◯without) the lateral side.

4. The prefix which makes typical mean NOT typical is (◯ab-, ◯ad-, ◯ a-, ◯ante-).

5. Adoral is (◯against, ◯before, ◯toward, ◯away from) the mouth.

III. FILL IN THE BLANK.
Using the word parts you have learned, enter the proper term in the space provided.

1. Remember that -emia means blood. Enter a word that means without enough blood or a low blood count. _____

2. Drawing toward the medial plane is _____ ducting.

3. Drawing away from the medial plane is _____ ducting.

4. If a condition warrants against doing something, that thing is _____ indicated.

5. A synonym for prenatal is _____.

Prefixes – Lesson 2 (Bi–Dy)

Following is a list of prefixes with their accompanying meanings and a sample word. Memorize these prefixes for the subsequent exercises.

Prefix	Meaning	Example
bi-/di-	two	bifid/dissect
brady-	slow	bradycardia
de-	down from, removing	decomposition
dia-	through, between, across	dialysis
dys-	difficult/abnormal	dysphagia

I. MATCHING.
Match the appropriate terms below.

1. ____ dys-

2. ____ de-

3. ____ bi-

4. ____ dia-

5. ____ brady-

A. down from

B. slow

C. difficult

D. two

E. across

II. TRUE/FALSE.
Mark the following true or false.

1. Bigeminy means occurring in sets of three.

   ○ true
   ○ false

2. The diameter is the length of the line passing through the center of the circle.

   ○ true
   ○ false

3. Dysmineralization is the removal of minerals.

   ○ true
   ○ false

4. Bradykinetic is characterized by fast movement.

   ○ true
   ○ false

5. Characterized by difficulty moving is dyskinetic.

   ○ true
   ○ false

III. FILL IN THE BLANK.
Using the word parts you have learned, enter the proper term in the space provided.

1. Pepsia is a word for digestion. Enter a word which means difficulty digesting.

   _____

2. Manual means done with the hands. Type a word which means done with two, or BOTH hands.

   _____

3. Hydration is the condition of being combined with water. Enter a word which means the removal of water from a substance or body. _____

4. Cardia is a word for the heart. _____ is slow heart (beat).

5. The medical name for diffuse perspiration is diaphoresis. This is because sweat emits profusely _____ the skin.

Prefixes – Lesson 3 (Ec–He)

Following is a list of prefixes with their accompanying meanings and a sample word. Memorize these prefixes for the subsequent exercises.

Prefix	Meaning	Example
ecto-/ex-/exo-	outside/without/away from	exophytic/ectoplasm
en-/endo-/em-/eso-	inside	encapsulated
epi-	above/on	epicondyle
eu-	good/normal	euthyroid
hemi-/semi-	half/partly	hemilaminectomy

I. MATCHING.
Match the appropriate terms below.

1. ____ hemi-
2. ____ ecto-
3. ____ epi-
4. ____ eu-
5. ____ endo-

A. above
B. good
C. half
D. inside
E. without/outside

II. TRUE/FALSE.
Mark the following true or false.

1. Endometrium is the outside of the mucous membrane.
   - ○ true
   - ○ false

2. Epitympanic means situated on the tympanum.
   - ○ true
   - ○ false

3. The ectoderm is the innermost layer of skin.
   - ○ true
   - ○ false

4. A hemiarthroplasty is a total formation of a joint.
   - ○ true
   - ○ false

5. Normal or proper mobility/movement is eukinesis.
   - ○ true
   - ○ false

III. FILL IN THE BLANK.
Using the word parts you have learned, enter the proper term in the space provided.

1. Menorrhea is a term for menstrual flow. _____ is normal menstrual flow.

2. _____ means situated upon the dura. (This requires an adjectival ending.)

3. Hale is Latin for breath. _____ means to breathe out.

4. Hemianopsia is blindness in _____ the visual field.

5. Cardia is heart. _____ means situated within the heart. (This requires an adjectival ending.)

Review: Lessons 1–3

I. **MATCHING.**
Match the appropriate terms below.

1. ____ anti-		A. toward
2. ____ dys-		B. no
3. ____ hemi-		C. against
4. ____ an-		D. slow
5. ____ de-		E. difficult
6. ____ ecto-		F. two
7. ____ dia-		G. inside
8. ____ ad-		H. half
9. ____ eu-		I. without/outside
10. ____ bi-		J. away from
11. ____ endo-		K. removing
12. ____ ab-		L. on
13. ____ epi-		M. through
14. ____ ante-		N. good
15. ____ brady-		O. before

II. **TRUE/FALSE.**
Mark the following true or false.

1. Antenatal means after birth.

   ◯ true
   ◯ false

2. An epicondyle is an eminence upon or above the condyle.

   ◯ true
   ◯ false

3. Encranial means situated outside the cranium.

   ◯ true
   ◯ false

4. Abduct means away from the medial plane.

   ○ true
   ○ false

5. Adduct means away from the medial plane.

   ○ true
   ○ false

6. Ectonuclear is outside the nucleus of a cell.

   ○ true
   ○ false

III. MULTIPLE CHOICE.
Choose the best answer.

1. A medicine which fights against or counteracts hypertension is an (○ahypertensive, ○ antehypertensive, ○antihypertensive) medication.

2. A slowed rhythm is (○birhythmia, ○bradyarrhythmia, ○dysrhythmia).

3. Lack or absence of symmetry is (○asymmetry, ○ansymmetry, ○antesymmetry).

4. (○Anticompression, ○Dyscompression, ○Decompression) is removal of pressure.

5. Hemiparesis is muscular weakness affecting (○all, ○half, ○none) of the body.

6. Bifurcated is divided into (○one, ○two, ○three) branches.

7. Dysphagia is (○difficulty, ○pain, ○absence of) swallowing.

8. An easy or painless death is the definition for (○epispadius, ○esophilia, ○euthanasia).

9. A diascope is an instrument pressed against the skin to see (○against, ○through, ○ upon) the skin.

IV. FILL IN THE BLANK.
Using the terms in the box, enter the correct term(s) in the space provided.

1. A term which means having two foci (plural of focus) is

   _____.

   (This word requires an adjectival ending.)

2. The point of separation between the stalk and the branch is the

   _____ physis.

3. Situated above the trochlea is _____.

4. Metri is the root word for uterus. Enter a word that means

   inflammation of the inner membrane of the uterus.

   _____

5. Enter a word for a substance that removes or reduces

   congestion. _____

6. Natal is an adjective for birth. Enter an adjective that means

   before birth. _____

7. A drug fighting against inflammation is an _____

   drug.

8. Phasia is a term denoting speech. Enter a word meaning difficult

   or abnormal speech. _____

9. In physical therapy adduction is moving _____ the

   medial plane.

10. In physical therapy abduction is moving _____ the

    medial plane.

11. A laminectomy is a kind of back surgery. Half a laminectomy is a

    _____.

12. Esthesia is sensation or feeling. Enter a word that means without

    or loss of feeling or sensation. _____

13. The _____ dermis is the outermost layer of three

    primary skin layers.

anesthesia
antenatal
anti-inflammatory
away from
bifocal
bradyarrhythmia
decongestant
dia
dysphasia
endometritis
epi
epitrochlear
eupnea
hemilaminectomy
toward

14. Pnea is breath. _____ is normal respiration.

15. Arrhythmia is an irregular heart rhythm. A slow irregular heart rhythm is _____.

Prefixes – Lesson 4 (Hy–In)

Following is a list of prefixes with their accompanying meanings and a sample word. Memorize these prefixes for the subsequent exercises.

Prefix	Meaning	Example
hyper-	excessive, greater than normal	hypercholesterolemia
hypo-/sub-	beneath/below normal, under	hyponatremia
in-	not	inability
infra-	beneath	infraorbital
inter-	between	intercondylar

I. **MATCHING.**
    Match the appropriate terms below.

1. ____ in-
2. ____ hypo-
3. ____ infra-
4. ____ hyper-
5. ____ inter-

A. excessive
B. between
C. below normal
D. beneath
E. not

II. **MULTIPLE CHOICE.**
     Choose the best answer.

1. Greater than normal cholesterol in the blood is (◯ hypocholesterol, ◯ hypocholesterolemia, ◯ hypercholesterolemia).

2. Situated under the tongue is (◯ inglossal, ◯ hypoglossal, ◯ hyperglossal).

3. Insubstantial means (◯not, ◯very, ◯excessively) substantial.

4. (◯Inter-, ◯Infra-, ◯In-) mammary is beneath the mammary glands.

5. Situated between the vertebrae would be (◯ infravertebral, ◯ intervertebral, ◯ subvertebral).

III. FILL IN THE BLANK.
Enter the correct word combination in the blank provided.

1. A prefix for between is _____ .

2. Infrascapular means situated _____ the scapula.

3. _____ is excessive activity.

4. Not active is _____ .

5. Glycemia is the concentration of glucose in the blood. Type a word for below normal concentration of glucose in the blood. _____ .

Prefixes – Lesson 5 (In–Mi)

Following is a list of prefixes with their accompanying meanings and a sample word. Memorize these prefixes for the subsequent exercises.

Prefix	Meaning	Example
intra-	within/inside of	intrauterine
macro-	large	macrosomia
mal-	bad	malalignment
meso-	middle or moderate	mesothelial
micro-	small	microhematuria

I. MATCHING.
Match the appropriate terms below.

1. ____ macro-
2. ____ meso-
3. ____ intra-
4. ____ mal-
5. ____ micro-

A. large
B. within
C. bad
D. small
E. middle

II. MULTIPLE CHOICE.
Choose the best answer.

1. Bad or improper alignment is (◯ macroalignment, ◯ mesoalignment, ◯ malalignment).

2. Intra-abdominal is (◯inside,◯between,◯above) the abdomen.

3. A microscope enables you to study (◯ small, ◯ large, ◯ bad) things.

4. Macromastia is having (◯ small, ◯ large, ◯ bad) breasts.

5. The middle layer of three primary germ layers of the embryo is the (◯ micro-, ◯ meso-, ◯ intra-) derm.

III. FILL IN THE BLANK.
Enter the correct word combination in the blank provided.

1. A tiny embolus would be a _____ .

2. Intraorbital means _____ the orbit.

3. Abnormal or bad rotation is _____ .

4. Mesophlebitis is inflammation of the _____ coat of a vein.

5. Macrognathia is a condition characterized by abnormally _____ jaws.

Prefixes – Lesson 6 (Mu–Pe)

Following is a list of prefixes with their accompanying meanings and a sample word. Memorize these prefixes for the subsequent exercises.

Prefix	Meaning	Example
multi-/poly-	many/excessive	multinodular/polyhydramnios
mono-/uni-	one	monochorionic/unilateral
nulli-	none	nulliparous
para-	near, beside, resembling, abnormal	parahepatic
per-	through, by, or completely	percutaneous

I. MATCHING.
Match the appropriate terms below.

1. ____ mono-

2. ____ per-

3. ____ multi-

4. ____ nulli-

5. ____ para-

A. many
B. through
C. none
D. near
E. one

II. TRUE/FALSE.
Mark the following true or false.

1. Nulliparous means never having given birth to a viable infant.
   - ○ true
   - ○ false

2. Paramedian is situated at the farthest point from the midline.
   - ○ true
   - ○ false

3. Monoclonal is derived from one cell.
   - ○ true
   - ○ false

4. Multinodular is characterized by one nodule.
   - ○ true
   - ⊙ false

5. Percutaneous means performed beside the skin.
   - ○ true
   - ○ false

III. FILL IN THE BLANK.
Enter the correct word combination in the blank provided.

1. Perforation is the act of boring _____ a part.

2. Inflammation near the appendix is _____ .

3. Dipsia means thirst. Enter a word meaning excessive thirst (needing many drinks).

   _____ .

4. Enter a word meaning having a single pole. _____

5. _____ means none.

Review: Lessons 4–6

I. MATCHING.
Match the appropriate terms below.

1. _____ intra-
2. _____ mal-
3. _____ hyper-
4. _____ multi-
5. _____ micro-
6. _____ per-
7. _____ in-
8. _____ macro-
9. _____ nulli-
10. _____ para-
11. _____ hypo-
12. _____ mono-
13. _____ infra-
14. _____ meso-
15. _____ inter-

A. within
B. excessive
C. many
D. not
E. bad
F. beside
G. below normal
H. one
I. large
J. beneath (positionally)
K. none
L. small
M. through
N. middle
O. between

II. MULTIPLE CHOICE.
Choose the correct answer.

1. Infraclavicular is (◯ between, ◯ through, ◯ beneath) the clavicle.

2. A vitamin pill which contains many vitamins is a (◯ multi-, ◯ nulli-, ◯ macro-) vitamin.

3. Intrauterine means (◯ between, ◯ within, ◯ underneath) the uterus.

4. Perfusion is a liquid poured (◯ through, ◯ around, ◯ beneath) an organ or tissue.

5. Microcardia is (◯ smallness, ◯ largeness, ◯ absence) of the heart.

6. Unicameral means having (◯ many, ◯ large, ◯ one) cavity or compartment.

7. Increase in the number of normal cells in a tissue is (○ hypo-, ○ hyper-, ○ mono-) plasia.

8. Connected or situated between two or more cartilages is (○ intracartilaginous, ○ hypocartilaginous, ○ intercartilaginous).

III. FILL IN THE BLANK.
Using the terms in the box, enter the correct term(s) in the space provided.

1. -Pnea means breath. _____ is an abnormal increase in depth and rate of inspiration.

2. Permeate means to pass _____ a filter.

3. Enter a word that means within the cranium.

   _____

4. Enter a word meaning having numerous lobes.

   _____

5. Having had no children is _____ parous.

6. Combine the terms meso- + theli/o + -al. _____

7. Create a word meaning bad absorption. _____

8. Mono- means _____.

9. Create a word meaning situated beneath the orbit (this requires an adjectival ending). _____

10. Situated near the liver (combining form hepat/o) would be _____. (This word is also an adjective.)

11. Hematuria means blood within the urine. Microhematuria means an extremely _____ amount of blood within the urine.

12. A word for not substantial is _____.

13. Interventricular means _____ the ventricles.

14. Macroadenoma is a _____ adenomatous tumor.

15. The word _____ means situated under the diaphragm.

between
hyperpnea
infradiaphragmatic
infraorbital
insubstantial
intracranial
large
malabsorption
mesothelial
multilobar
nulli
one
parahepatic
small
through

IV. TRUE/FALSE.
Mark the following true or false.

1. Maladjusted means well or normally adjusted.

   ○ true
   ○ false

2. Paraumbilical means between the umbilicus.

   ○ true
   ○ false

3. Nulli- means much.

   ○ true
   ○ false

4. Inability means NOT able.

   ○ true
   ○ false

5. Percutaneous means through the skin.

   ○ true
   ○ false

6. Mesonasal means situated beneath the nose.

   ○ true
   ○ false

7. Macrosomatia means great bodily size.

   ○ true
   ○ false

Prefixes – Lesson 7 (Pe–Re)

Following is a list of prefixes with their accompanying meanings and a sample word. Memorize these prefixes for the subsequent exercises.

Prefix	Meaning	Example
peri-	around/near	periventricular
post-	after, behind	postoperative
primi-	first	primigravida
re-	back, again	redo
retro-	behind, backward	retroareolar

I. MATCHING.
Match the prefix with the appropriate meaning below.

1. ____ post-
2. ____ re-
3. ____ peri-
4. ____ retro-
5. ____ primi-

A. after
B. first
C. backward
D. around
E. again

II. MULTIPLE CHOICE.
Choose the correct answer.

1. Periappendicitis means inflammation (◯beneath, ◯behind, ◯around) the appendix.

2. A reanastomosis is an anastomosis that is performed (◯for the first time, ◯again, ◯never) .

3. Retroareolar means situated (◯around, ◯behind, ◯underneath) the areola.

4. (◯Pre-, ◯Post-, ◯Peri-) operative means after the operation.

5. Primigravida means pregnant for the (◯first, ◯second, ◯last) time.

III. FILL IN THE BLANK.
Using the word parts you have learned, enter the proper term in the space provided.

1. The prefix retro- means _____ .

2. Tonsillar is an adjective meaning pertaining to a tonsil. Type a word that means situated around a tonsil. _____

3. Primary pertains to the _____ in order.

4. Postictal means _____ a stroke or epileptic seizure.

5. Reactivate is to make active _____ .

Prefixes – Lesson 8 (Su–Un)

Following is a list of prefixes with their accompanying meanings and a sample word. Memorize these prefixes for the subsequent exercises.

Prefix	Meaning	Example
super-	more than normal, excessive	superinfection

supra-	above, over		suprapubic
sy(n)(m)-	together, union		symphysis
tachy-	fast		tachyarrhythmia
trans-	across/through		transesophageal
uni-	one		unilateral

I. MATCHING.
Match the prefix with the appropriate meaning below.

1. ____ tachy-

2. ____ trans-

3. ____ uni-

4. ____ supra-

5. ____ syn-

6. ____ super-

A. excessive
B. together
C. fast
D. across
E. one
F. above

II. TRUE/FALSE.
Mark the following true or false.

1. Suprapubic means situated above the pubis.
   ○ true
   ○ false

2. Tachyarrhythmia is defined as a slower than normal rhythm.
   ○ true
   ○ false

3. Unipolar means having but one pole.
   ○ true
   ○ false

4. Supermotility is slow movement.
   ○ true
   ○ false

5. Symbiosis in parasitology is two dissimilar organisms living in union with one another.

○ true
○ false

6. Transtracheal means underneath the trachea.

○ true
○ false

III. FILL IN THE BLANK.
Using the word parts you have learned, enter the proper term in the space provided.

1. Flowing in only one direction is _____ directional.

2. Symplastic is marked by _____ of protoplasm.

3. An abnormally fast heartbeat is called _____ cardia.

4. Transesophageal means _____ the esophagus.

5. Suprachoroid means situated _____ the choroid.

6. Abnormally increased sensitivity is _____ sensitivity.

Prefixes – Lesson 9 (Sound-Alikes)

One problem encountered in medical transcription editing is words that are pronounced the same or sound very similar, but that are spelled differently. As a medical transcription editor, you will notice that this is a recurring problem. That is why it is SO important to learn the different meanings and be able to differentiate between the different spellings in these cases.

Inter-/Intra-

This is one example of the above-mentioned problem. Most dictating doctors do not say words slowly enough for the speech recognition program to distinguish a difference in the sounds. These prefixes are used with such frequency that they are rarely enunciated clearly, and they end up sounding the same. The meanings for inter- and intra- are so different that you can learn to assess which one is appropriate by the context.

For example, a common mistake among new medical transcription editors is to not recognize that words like *interabdominal, interuterine,* and *intercranial* are incorrect. You should notice that these words would mean BETWEEN the two abdomens, BETWEEN the two uteri, and BETWEEN the two heads! This is, of course, anatomically impossible—as no one has two of these structures (or at least most people!). In order for the prefix inter- to be appropriate, there MUST be TWO or more of whatever structure is being referred to. Therefore, the correct usage in these cases is the prefix intra-, meaning WITHIN the abdomen, uterus, or cranium.

By the same token, the prefix inter- is used correctly in such words as *intervertebral* (between the vertebrae), *interventricular* (between the ventricles), and *intertrochanteric* (between the trochanters). And, because things are always more complicated than they need to be, there are words that can take either prefix—*intermedullary/intramedullary* or *interventricular/intraventricular*.

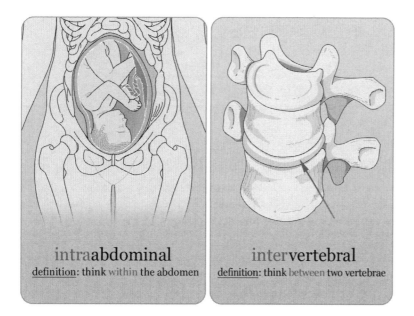

intraabdominal
definition: think within the abdomen

intervertebral
definition: think between two vertebrae

There are, of course, instances in which either prefix could be used. At first, you must listen carefully and try to distinguish a difference in sounds. You can also look up both possibilities in the dictionary. However, often all possible prefix and suffix combinations for a particular root will not be found in the dictionary. In these cases, there is usually one prefix that consistently goes with a certain root word or term. It will be necessary for you to determine, by asking an experienced medical transcription editor or by trial and error, which prefix is correct, and memorize it.

Super-/Supra-

Another example of the same problem is supra-/super-. Spoken rapidly, these sound the same and are difficult to distinguish, except by context. Again, you need to understand the meanings of both of these prefixes. After you have done a few, you can learn which words generally go with each prefix. For example, you are likely to hear *superimposition* and *suprapubic*. One means imposed over the whole or an excessive part, and the other means located above. Some other examples are *suprahyoid, supermotility, and superficial*.

Peri-/Para-

It is very difficult to distinguish between these two prefixes in regular dictation, as they are both said so quickly and sound similar. However, these two prefixes present a unique problem: they also have very similar meanings. In fact, generally speaking, the two can be used interchangeably. You will need to train yourself to try to hear exactly which one the dictator is using. However, there are some words that require one or the other and are incorrect if the wrong prefix is used. For example, *perianal*. A rule that is sometimes helpful in distinguishing between peri/para is to think of para as parallel to and peri as around. So if the structure referred to is long and/or tubular, use para: *paraspinal, paratracheal, paraesophageal*. If the structure is more rounded or compact, use peri: *periumbilical, perihilar, perinephric*.

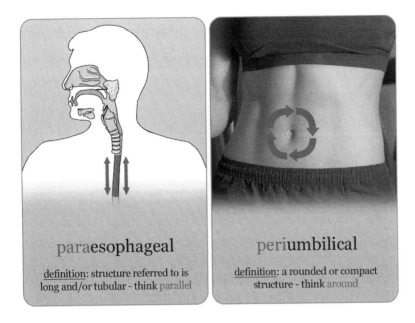

paraesophageal

definition: structure referred to is long and/or tubular - think parallel

periumbilical

definition: a rounded or compact structure - think around

Ab-/Ad-

This is another set of prefixes that sound virtually the same when dictated. The root word that accompanies these prefixes is commonly -duct, as in *abduct* and *adduct*. Often dictators will say the letters individually because it is so difficult to distinguish the difference in pronunciation. For example: A-D duct or A-B duct. Remember, *abnormal* is "away from" normal and you can easily identify meaning when necessary.

Prefixes – Lesson 10 (Synonymous Prefixes)

You probably noticed that there are some prefixes that share the same meaning. For example "away from" is a definition for ab- as well as ecto-/ex-/exo-. As a medical transcription editor, the important thing is to be able to spell the prefixes correctly and be sure that they form appropriate words. Remember, it will not be your responsibility to create words out of the blue or strictly from definitions. You will ALWAYS hear them FIRST. However, the more you know, the better qualified you are to make judgment calls and the better editor you will make.

The following review exercises will, therefore, contain problems for which more than one answer will be possible. Try to determine ALL correct answers for a definition. Also, looking up a word in the dictionary or word list will enable you to better learn the new word and determine which prefix is preferred for that particular meaning.

I. MATCHING.
In this exercise, every prefix has one correct definition. Choose the *best* answer.

1. ____ macro-
2. ____ dys-
3. ____ peri-
4. ____ inter-
5. ____ hemi-
6. ____ ad-
7. ____ ecto-
8. ____ intra-
9. ____ mal-
10. ____ super-
11. ____ tachy-
12. ____ para-
13. ____ anti-
14. ____ ab-
15. ____ brady-
16. ____ meso-
17. ____ retro-
18. ____ post-
19. ____ primi-
20. ____ supra-

A. backward
B. large
C. above, over
D. around
E. first
F. toward
G. half, partly
H. slow
I. fast
J. difficult
K. out/without/outside
L. within
M. bad
N. away from
O. after
P. excessive
Q. against
R. middle
S. near, beside
T. between

II. MULTIPLE ANSWER.
Choose the applicable answer(s).

1. Select the two prefixes with the definition of abnormal.

   ☐ mal-
   ☐ anti-
   ☐ para-
   ☐ ecto-
   ☐ dys-
   ☐ retro-

2. Select the three prefixes with the definition of beneath or under.

   ☐ hypo-
   ☐ dys-
   ☐ sub-
   ☐ ad-
   ☐ mal-
   ☐ infra-

3. Select the two prefixes with the definition of above.

   ☐ inter-
   ☐ para-
   ☐ epi-
   ☐ supra-
   ☐ post-
   ☐ super-

4. Select the two prefixes with the definition of between.

   ☐ inter-
   ☐ anti-
   ☐ supra-
   ☐ dia-
   ☐ hemi-
   ☐ peri-

III. MULTIPLE CHOICE.
Choose the best answer.

1. A procedure which is performed through the skin is (◯per-, ◯peri-, ◯para-) cutaneous.

2. Abnormally slow movement is (◯tachy-, ◯brady-) kinesis.

3. The cervix of a woman who has never given birth is (◯nulli-, ◯primi-, ◯poly-) parous.

4. Occurring within the heart is (◯ ex-, ◯ endo-, ◯ exo-) cardial.

5. A patient is taken to recovery from surgery (◯ pre-, ◯ post-) operatively.

6. If there is surgical removal of only half of a vertebral lamina it is called a (◯ primi-, ◯ hemi-, ◯ retro-) laminectomy.

IV. TRUE/FALSE.
Mark the following true or false.

1. Taking place before an operation is preoperative.

   ◯ true
   ◯ false

2. Under the diaphragm is interdiaphragmatic.

   ◯ true
   ◯ false

3. Normal or good nutrition is malnutrition.

   ◯ true
   ◯ false

4. Retro-orbital means behind the orbit.

   ◯ true
   ◯ false

5. Anechoic means without echoes.

   ◯ true
   ◯ false

Review: Lessons 7–10

I. MATCHING.
Match the prefix with the appropriate meaning below.

1. ____ peri-

2. ____ para-

3. ____ syn-

4. ____ tachy-

5. ____ inter-

6. ____ uni-

7. ____ supra-

8. ____ super-

9. ____ post-

10. ____ re-

11. ____ intra-

12. ____ retro-

13. ____ primi-

14. ____ hypo-

A. after
B. union
C. excessive
D. backward
E. within
F. first
G. around
H. again
I. above
J. between
K. fast
L. beside
M. one
N. below normal

II. MULTIPLE CHOICE.
Choose the correct answer.

1. If one has diminished glucose in the blood, he/she has (◯hyper-, ◯hypo-) glycemia.

2. If one has an excess of calcium in the blood, he/she has (◯hyper-, ◯hypo-) calcemia.

3. The ultrasound shows an (◯intra-, ◯inter-) uterine gestation.

4. Incomplete or underdevelopment of an organ or tissue is (◯hyper-, ◯hypo-) plasia.

5. Situated between the malleoli would be (◯inter-, ◯intra-) malleolar.

6. Tachyarrhythmia is (◯slow, ◯fast, ◯no) rhythm.

7. A woman who has had one pregnancy that resulted in a live-born fetus would be considered (◯primipara, ◯multipara).

8. (◯Re-, ◯Post-) anastomose is to create a connection between two structures again.

9. Retrograde is moving (◯around, ◯backward, ◯together) or against the usual direction.

10. Postauricular is located (◯behind, ◯around, ◯above) the auricle of the ear.

11. Unicameral is having (◯one, ◯zero) cavities or compartments.

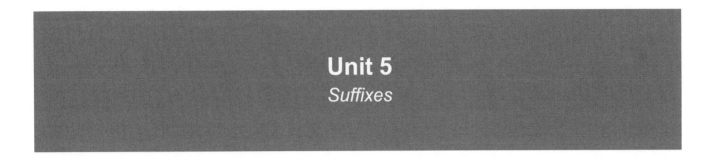

Unit 5
Suffixes

Suffixes – Introduction

The final category of word parts we will be presenting is suffixes. We saved these for last because they are typically the easiest to identify. The lessons, exercises, and tests in this unit cover suffixes that begin with A and continue through suffixes that begin with T.

- *Suffixes A–M in Lessons 1–6*
- *Suffixes O–T in Lessons 7–11*
- *Synonymous Suffixes in Lesson 12*

Some of the suffixes create adjectives and others create nouns. It is important to learn the adjectival endings well, because you may be required to identify adjectives, for several reasons, in medical reports. This will make that job easier. Also, for the remainder of the program you will see many definitions and be required to build many words that employ adjectival endings. We will begin our study of suffixes with those beginning with A–M.

Suffixes – Lesson 1 (Ab–Ce)

Following is a list of suffixes with their accompanying meanings and a sample word. Memorize these suffixes for the subsequent exercises.

Suffixes	Meaning	Example
-able/-ible*	capable of	remarkable
-ac/-al/-an/-ar/-ary/-eal/-ic/-ive/-tic*	pertaining to	fundal/ pancreatic
-ase	enzyme	amylase
-algia	pain	myalgia
-cele	hernia (protrusion of organ through its containing wall)	cystocele

The above suffixes change the part of speech they are attached to from a noun to an adjective.

Some of the suffixes listed above create adjectives and other nouns. It is important to learn the adjectival endings well, because you may be required to identify adjectives, for several reasons, in medical reports. This will make that job easier.

I. MULTIPLE CHOICE.
Identify which words are adjectives and which are nouns by determining the meaning.

1. -algia
   - ○ adjective
   - ○ noun

2. -ible
   - ○ adjective
   - ○ noun

3. -ive
   - ○ adjective
   - ○ noun

4. -ase
   - ○ adjective
   - ○ noun

5. -eal
   - ○ adjective
   - ○ noun

6. -ary
   - ○ adjective
   - ○ noun

7. -cele
   - ○ adjective
   - ○ noun

8. -al
   - ○ adjective
   - ○ noun

9. -able
   - ○ adjective
   - ○ noun

10. -tic/-ic
    - ○ adjective
    - ○ noun

II. MATCHING.
Match the suffixes with their correct meanings.

1. ____ -cele
2. ____ -algia
3. ____ -ase
4. ____ -ary
5. ____ -ible

A. enzyme
B. capable of
C. hernia
D. pain
E. pertaining to

III. MULTIPLE CHOICE.
Select the correct answer. If there is more than one correct answer, just choose one.

1. The suffix which means hernia is _____.
   - ○ -cele
   - ○ -able
   - ○ -ase
   - ○ -ic

2. The suffix which means pertaining to is _____.
   - ○ -ible
   - ○ -ic
   - ○ -ase
   - ○ -eal

3. The suffix which means pain is _____.
   - ○ -ary
   - ○ -ase
   - ○ -algia
   - ○ -eal

4. This means capable of.
   - ○ -cele
   - ○ -algia
   - ○ -ible
   - ○ -able

5. An ending for enzyme is _____.
   - ○ -ar
   - ○ -al
   - ○ -ase
   - ○ -ary

IV. FILL IN THE BLANK.

Enter the correct word in the blank provided. If necessary, it is acceptable to consult a dictionary or your word list to determine which of several suffixes would be the preferred one.

1. Compress means press together; enter a word which means capable of being pressed together.

   _____

2. Arthr/o is the combining form for joint; enter a word that means pain in the joint.

   _____

3. The suffix -ase means _____ .

4. If cyst/o means bladder, then a protrusion of the bladder through its wall would be a

   _____ .

5. Appendic/o is the combining form for appendix; enter a word which means pertaining to the appendix. _____

Suffixes – Lesson 2 (Ce–Em)

Following is a list of suffixes with their accompanying meanings and a sample word. Memorize these suffixes for the subsequent exercises.

Suffixes	Meaning	Example
-centesis	procedure to aspirate fluid	paracentesis
-ectasia/-ectasis	dilation	telangiectasia
-ectomy	excision or removal	appendectomy
-edema	swelling	lymphedema
-emesis	vomiting	hematemesis

I. MATCHING.
Match the appropriate terms below.

1. ____ -edema
2. ____ -centesis
3. ____ -ectasis
4. ____ -emesis
5. ____ -ectomy

A. swelling
B. dilation
C. excision or removal
D. procedure to aspirate fluid
E. vomiting

II. MULTIPLE CHOICE.
Choose the correct answer.

1. A suffix meaning dilation is (○-centesis, ○-ectomy, ○-ectasia, ○-emesis).

2. Swelling is (○-edema, ○-emesis. ○-ectasis, ○-ectasia).

3. (○-Emesis, ○-Centesis, ○-Cele, ○-Ectomy) is a procedure to aspirate fluid.

4. Excision or removal is the meaning of the suffix (○-edema, ○-ectasis, ○-centesis, ○-ectomy).

5. A suffix which means vomiting is (○-ectasis, ○-edema, ○-emesis, ○-ectasia).

III. FILL IN THE BLANK.
Using the word parts you have learned, enter the proper term in the space provided.

1. Atel/o is a combining form which means imperfect. A word meaning imperfect dilation, then, would be _____.

2. Append/i is the combining form for appendix. Removal of the appendix would be

   _____.

3. If hemat/o means blood, then _____ means vomiting up blood.

4. A procedure to aspirate amniotic fluid would be called an _____.

5. Edema is a word for _____.

Suffixes – Lesson 3 (Em–Gr)

Following is a list of suffixes with their accompanying meanings and a sample word. Memorize these suffixes for the subsequent exercises.

Suffixes	Meaning	Example
-emia	blood	anemia
-genic/-genesis*	beginning/producing	osteogenic
-gram	record	cholangiogram
-graph	instrument for recording	polygraph
-graphy	process of recording	echocardiography

*This suffix has an adjectival ending

I. MATCHING.
Match the appropriate terms below.

1. _____ -graph
2. _____ -emia
3. _____ -genesis
4. _____ -gram
5. _____ -graphy

A. record
B. process of recording
C. blood
D. beginning
E. instrument

II. MULTIPLE CHOICE.
Choose the best answer.

1. The suffix meaning blood is (○ -emesis, ○ -emia, ○ -ectasis, ○ -edema).

2. (○ -Graph, ○ -Graphy, ○ -Genesis, ○ -Gram) means beginning.

3. An instrument is a (○ -graph, ○ -gram, ○ -graphy).

4. The process of recording is (○ -graph, ○ -gram, ○ -graphy).

5. A record is (○ -graph, ○ -gram, ○ -graphy).

III. FILL IN THE BLANK.
Using the word parts you have learned, enter the proper term in the space provided.

1. The meaning of -emia is _____.

2. If cardi/o means heart, then a record of a heart tracing would be a _____.

3. Likewise, the technique for recording the heart would be _____.

4. And finally, the instrument for recording the heart tracing would be called a _____.

5. Oste/o is the combining form for bone. _____ is the formation of bone.

Review: Lessons 1–3

I. **MATCHING.**
   Match the appropriate terms below.

1. ____ -centesis

2. ____ -ase

3. ____ -ectasia

4. ____ -algia

5. ____ -emia

6. ____ -graph

7. ____ -ectomy

8. ____ -ible

9. ____ -graphy

10. ____ -edema

11. ____ -genesis

12. ____ -gram

13. ____ -cele

14. ____ -emesis

15. ____ -ary

A. hernia
B. swelling
C. capable of
D. beginning/production
E. vomiting
F. enzyme
G. process of recording
H. pain
I. dilation
J. pertaining to
K. record
L. procedure to aspirate fluid
M. blood
N. excision or removal
O. instrument for recording

II. FILL IN THE BLANK.
Using the terms in the box, enter the correct term(s) in the space provided.

1. Enter the word amni/o + -centesis. _____

2. Amni/o is a root that refers to the sac surrounding the fetus. Centesis means _____.

3. An appendectomy is _____ of the appendix.

4. Diction refers to a choice of words. A book pertaining to words is a _____.

5. Hypoglycemia is an abnormally diminished amount of glucose in the _____.

6. Rect/o is a combining form meaning rectum. Enter a word that means a rectal hernia. _____

7. My/o is a combining form meaning muscle. Myalgia is _____ in the muscle.

8. Hyper means excessive or increased. A term for excessive vomiting would be _____. (Hyper- is a prefix. In this particular word, -emesis functions as the root.)

9. Combine the following roots: ech/o + cardi/o + -gram.

   _____

10. Lipase is a kind of _____.

11. Cry/o means cold. A word pertaining to the producing of cold temperatures would be _____.

amniocentesis
blood
cryogenic
dictionary
echocardiogram
enzyme
excision
hyperemesis
pain
procedure to aspirate fluid
rectocele

Suffixes – Lesson 4 (I)

Following is a list of suffixes with their accompanying meanings and a sample word. Memorize these suffixes for the subsequent exercises.

Suffixes	Meaning	Example
-ia/-iasis	condition	psoriasis
-ism	condition	botulism
-ist	one who	psychologist
-itis	inflammation	pancreatitis

I. MATCHING.
Match the appropriate terms below.

1. ____ -ist
2. ____ -ia
3. ____ -iasis
4. ____ -ism
5. ____ -itis

A. condition
B. one who
C. inflammation

II. MULTIPLE CHOICE.
Choose the correct answer.

1. A suffix meaning inflammation is (◯ -ism, ◯ -itis, ◯ -ist).

2. Which of the following does NOT mean condition? (◯ -iasis, ◯ -ism, ◯ -itis).

3. Inflammation of the pancreas is called pancreat (◯-itis, ◯-ism, ◯-ist).

4. An (◯-ia/-iasis, ◯-itis, ◯-ist) is one who.

III. TRUE/FALSE.
Mark the following true or false.

1. If a word ends in -ist we are talking about a person.
   ◯ true
   ◯ false

2. Psoriasis and botulism are examples of two different suffixes that have the same meaning.
   ◯ true
   ◯ false

3. -ia means condition.
   ◯ true
   ◯ false

4. -itis means inflammation.
   ◯ true
   ◯ false

Suffixes – Lesson 5 (Ki–Ly)

Following is a list of suffixes with their accompanying meanings and a sample word. Memorize these suffixes for the subsequent exercises.

Suffixes	Meaning	Example
-kinesia/-kinesis	movement/motion	hypokinesis
-logist	specialist	radiologist
-logy	study of	pathology
-lysis	loosening/freeing/breaking apart/destroying	adhesiolysis
-lytic*	pertaining to destruction	hemolytic

Note the adjectival ending attached to this suffix. When determining which of the two suffixes, -lysis or -lytic, is the appropriate answer, decide if the word it creates is a noun or an adjective. Remember, -tic/-ic is the ending which means "pertaining to" or "characterized by" and it is the adjectival ending. Thus, if the suffix is "lysis," the term is a noun; if it is "lytic," the term is an adjective. For example: the process of breaking down into its component parts is "analysis." Pertaining to breaking down into its component parts is "analytic."

I. MATCHING.
Match the appropriate terms below.

1. ____ -lytic
2. ____ -kinesia/-kinesis
3. ____ -lysis
4. ____ -logy
5. ____ -logist

A. study of
B. loosening/freeing
C. specialist
D. pertaining to destruction
E. movement/motion

II. MULTIPLE CHOICE.
Choose the best answer.

1. The study of bones would end in (◯-lytic, ◯-logy, ◯-lysis).

2. The destruction or dissolution of bone would be osteo- (◯-lytic, ◯-lysis, ◯-logist).

3. The surgical freeing of adhesions would utilize the suffix (◯-lysis, ◯-logist, ◯-kinesia).

4. Hypokinesis is a word dealing with (◯ inflammation, ◯ specialist, ◯ movement).

5. A (◯ pathologist, ◯ radiology, ◯ neonatology) is a disease specialist.

III. FILL IN THE BLANK.
Using the word parts you have learned, enter the proper term in the space provided.

1. "Dys" means abnormal. Create a word that means abnormal movement or motion.

   _____

2. "Bio" means life. What would the study of life be? _____

3. "Spondylo" means vertebra. _____ would be dissolution or destruction of a vertebra.

4. A gastroenterologist is a doctor who _____ in disorders of the gastrointestinal tract.

Suffixes – Lesson 6 (M)

Following is a list of suffixes with their accompanying meanings and a sample word. Memorize these suffixes for the subsequent exercises.

Suffix	Meaning	Example
-malacia	softening	chondromalacia
-mania	preoccupation	pyromania
-megaly	enlargement	cardiomegaly
-meter	instrument to measure	glucometer
-metry	process of measuring	geometry

I. MATCHING.
Match the appropriate terms below.

1. ____ -mania
2. ____ -meter
3. ____ -megaly
4. ____ -malacia
5. ____ -metry

A. enlargement
B. process of measuring
C. preoccupation
D. softening
E. instrument to measure

II. FILL IN THE BLANK.
Using the word parts you have learned, enter the proper term in the space provided.

1. Chondromalacia is the _____ of cartilage.

2. Flowmetry would be a _____ .

3. Hepatomegaly is the _____ of the liver.

4. Preoccupation with oneself is ego-_____ .

5. A thermo-_____ is used to measure temperature.

III. TRUE/FALSE.
Mark the following true or false.

1. A preoccupation with fire is pyrometer.

   ○ true
   ○ false

2. Splenomegaly means enlargement of the spleen.

   ○ true
   ○ false

3. Malacia means softening.

   ○ true
   ○ false

4. A glucometer is an instrument to measure glucose.

   ○ true
   ○ false

5. -Metry is a suffix meaning complicated mathematical system.

   ○ true
   ○ false

Review: Lessons 4–6

I. **MATCHING.**
   Match the appropriate terms below. Some terms may be used more than once.

1. ____ -megaly
2. ____ -metry
3. ____ -ia/iasis
4. ____ -logy
5. ____ -ist
6. ____ -malacia
7. ____ -lysis
8. ____ -kinesia/-kinesis
9. ____ -ism
10. ____ -mania
11. ____ -meter
12. ____ -lytic
13. ____ -itis
14. ____ -logist

A. softening
B. process of measuring
C. study of
D. condition
E. pertaining to destruction
F. preoccupation
G. movement/motion
H. instrument to measure
I. specialist
J. inflammation
K. enlargement
L. loosening/breaking apart/freeing
M. one who

II. FILL IN THE BLANK.
Using the terms in the box, enter the correct term(s) in the space provided.

1. The study of the heart is _____.

2. An oxi_____ is used to measure the oxygen saturation.

3. Duodenitis is _____ of the duodenum.

4. Giardiasis is a _____ caused by the bacteria giardia.

5. An x-ray of the chest might demonstrate cardiomegaly, or _____ of the heart.

6. If a patient is preoccupied with something, he has a _____ about it.

7. Malacia is a _____.

8. A urologist is a _____.

9. Brady- is a prefix meaning slow. Abnormally slow movement would be _____.

bradykinesia
cardiology
condition
enlargement
inflammation
mania
meter
softening
specialist in urology

Suffixes – Lesson 7 (Oi–Os)

Following is a list of suffixes with their accompanying meanings and a sample word. Memorize these suffixes for the subsequent exercises.

Suffixes	Meaning	Example
-oid	resembling	adenoid
-oma	tumor	lymphoma
-opia	vision	diplopia
-ose	sugar	glucose
-osis	condition*	ptosis

This particular meaning of condition is usually abnormal; in particular, it means proliferation or an increased number of. For example: a diverticulum is a process in the abdomen. If there are several diverticula present, the patient is said to have diverticulosis.

I. MATCHING.
Match the appropriate terms below.

1. ___ -opia
2. ___ -oid
3. ___ -osis
4. ___ -oma
5. ___ -ose

A. vision
B. sugar
C. tumor
D. condition
E. resembling

II. FILL IN THE BLANK.
Using the word parts you have learned, enter the proper term in the space provided.

1. If a patient has myopia, it is a problem pertaining to his _____.

2. Fructose is a _____.

3. A glioblastoma is a kind of _____.

4. A lesion that resembles mucus would be a _____ lesion.

5. Nephrosis is a _____ affecting the kidneys.

III. TRUE/FALSE.
Mark the following true or false.

1. Glucose is a condition.
   ○ true
   ○ false

2. A carcinoma is a tumor.
   ○ true
   ○ false

3. Mycosis is a condition.
   ○ true
   ○ false

4. Diplopia is a condition of the feet.

   ○ true
   ○ false

5. Dermoid means resembling skin.

   ○ true
   ○ false

Suffixes – Lesson 8 (Ou–Ph)

Following is a list of suffixes with their accompanying meanings and a sample word. Memorize these suffixes for the subsequent exercises.

Suffixes	Meaning	Example
-ous	pertaining to/ characterized by	mucous
-pathy	disease or abnormality	adenopathy
-penia	deficiency	osteopenia
-pexy	surgical fixation	cystopexy
-phagia/-gic/-gy	eating/swallowing	dysphagia

I. **MATCHING.**
   Match the appropriate terms below.

   1. ____ -penia
   2. ____ -pathy
   3. ____ -phagia
   4. ____ -ous
   5. ____ -pexy

   A. eating/swallowing
   B. disease
   C. pertaining to
   D. deficiency
   E. surgical fixation

II. **FILL IN THE BLANK.**
    Using the word parts you have learned, enter the proper term in the space provided.

    1. If dys- is painful or abnormal, then dysphagia would be painful _____.

    2. Leukopenia would be a _____ of leukocytes in the blood.

    3. Something that is characterized by adenoma would be _____.

4. An orchiopexy would be a _____ of a testicle.

5. _____ is a suffix that means disease.

III. TRUE/FALSE.
Mark the following true or false.

1. Osteopenia is a deficiency of bone.

   ○ true
   ○ false

2. -Ous is a suffix that has to do with surgery.

   ○ true
   ○ false

3. Myelopathy employs a suffix that means diseased or pathological.

   ○ true
   ○ false

4. The suffix -pexy means surgical fixation.

   ○ true
   ○ false

5. Odynophagia is a word dealing with walking.

   ○ true
   ○ false

Suffixes – Lesson 9 (Ph–Rr)

Following is a list of suffixes with their accompanying meanings and a sample word. Memorize these suffixes for the subsequent exercises.

Suffixes	Meaning	Example
-phasia	speech	dysphasia
-phobia	abnormal fear	agoraphobia
-plasty	surgical repair	arthroplasty
-plegia	paralysis	paraplegia
-rrhage/-rrhagia	excessive flow or discharge	hemorrhage

I. MATCHING.
Match the appropriate terms below.

1. ____ -rrhagia
2. ____ -phasia
3. ____ -plasty
4. ____ -phobia
5. ____ -plegia

A. speech
B. abnormal fear
C. excessive flow or discharge
D. paralysis
E. surgical repair

II. FILL IN THE BLANK.
Using the word parts you have learned, enter the proper term in the space provided.

1. Using the prefix "a-," which means not, create a word that means inability to speak properly.

   _____

2. If a patient has severe arthritis, he may have an arthro_____, or a surgical repair of the joint.

3. A wound or organ that is hemorrhaging is one that is _____.

4. Quadriplegia utilizes the suffix meaning _____.

5. If you had a phobia about something, it would mean that you were _____ of it. (Think of claustrophobia).

III. TRUE/FALSE.
Mark the following true or false.

1. If a person is afflicted with aphasia, he has an abnormal fear of something.
   ○ true
   ○ false

2. A tympanoplasty would be the surgical repair of the tympanic membrane.
   ○ true
   ○ false

3. -Plegia means speech.
   ○ true
   ○ false

4. Hemophobia would be fear of bleeding or blood.

○ true
○ false

5. Hemorrhage would be fear of bleeding.

○ true
○ false

Review: Lessons 7–9

I. **MATCHING.**
Match the appropriate terms below.

1. ____ -osis
2. ____ -pexy
3. ____ -phagia/phagic
4. ____ -plasty
5. ____ -penia
6. ____ -ose
7. ____ -opia
8. ____ -phasia
9. ____ -pathy
10. ____ -oma
11. ____ -rrhage/-rrhagia
12. ____ -oid
13. ____ -plegia
14. ____ -ous
15. ____ -phobia

A. vision
B. speech
C. excessive flow or discharge
D. resembling
E. characterized by
F. deficiency
G. surgical repair
H. paralysis
I. tumor
J. surgical fixation
K. condition
L. sugar
M. eating/swallowing
N. abnormal fear
O. disease

II. TRUE/FALSE.
Mark the following true or false.

1. -Plasty is surgical repair.

   ◯ true
   ◯ false

2. -Pexy is surgical repair.

   ◯ true
   ◯ false

3. -Pexy is surgical fixation.

   ◯ true
   ◯ false

4. -Phasia and -phagia mean the same thing.

   ◯ true
   ◯ false

5. -Ose indicates an enzyme.

   ◯ true
   ◯ false

6. Lymphoid means resembling a lymph node.

   ◯ true
   ◯ false

7. Neurosis is a condition.

   ◯ true
   ◯ false

8. Osteopathy indicates a paralysis of some kind.

   ◯ true
   ◯ false

9. -Penia indicates an overabundance or hyperproduction of something, such as calcium.

   ◯ true
   ◯ false

10. Presbyopia is a term that has something to do with vision.

    ◯ true
    ◯ false

Suffixes – Lesson 10 (Rr–Sc)

Following is a list of suffixes with their accompanying meanings and a sample word. Memorize these suffixes for the subsequent exercises.

Suffixes	Meaning	Example
-rrhaphy	suture	herniorrhaphy
-rrhea	flow or discharge	diarrhea
-rrhexis	rupture	capsulorrhexis
-sclerosis	hardening	atherosclerosis
-scopy	examination with an instrument	colonoscopy

I. **MATCHING.**
   Match the appropriate terms below.

   1. ____ -rrhexis
   2. ____ -scopy
   3. ____ -sclerosis
   4. ____ -rrhaphy
   5. ____ -rrhea

   A. flow or discharge
   B. rupture
   C. suture
   D. hardening
   E. examination with an instrument

II. **FILL IN THE BLANK.**
   Enter the correct word combination in the blank provided.

   1. Atherosclerosis is _____ of the arteries.

   2. -Rrhexis means _____ .

   3. Endoscopy, cystoscopy, arthroscopy, etc. are examples of when a patient is _____ with an 4._____ .

   5. The suturing of a hernia (combining form herni/o) is _____ .

   6. Gonorrhea utilizes a suffix which means _____ .

III. TRUE/FALSE.
Mark the following true or false.

1. A laryngoscopy would be an examination of the larynx.

   ○ true
   ○ false

2. The suffix meaning hardening is -rrhexis.

   ○ true
   ○ false

3. If men/o is a combining form denoting relationship to the menses, then menorrhea would refer to the flow or discharge of menstruation.

   ○ true
   ○ false

4. There are not any suffixes which could appropriately be used to mean suture.

   ○ true
   ○ false

5. -Sclerosis means softening.

   ○ true
   ○ false

Suffixes – Lesson 11 (Sp–Tr)

Following is a list of suffixes with their accompanying meanings and a sample word. Memorize these suffixes for the subsequent exercises.

Suffixes	Meaning	Example
-spasm	twitching	bronchospasm
-stasis	stopping	hemostasis
-stomy	forming of an opening	tracheostomy
-tome	an instrument for cutting	osteotome
-tomy	incision (cutting into)	craniotomy
-tripsy	surgical crushing	lithotripsy
-trophic*/-trophy	nutrition	hypertrophy

*When placed with a root, -trophic creates an adjective.

I. MATCHING.
Match the appropriate terms below.

1. ____ -tome
2. ____ -spasm
3. ____ -stasis
4. ____ -stomy
5. ____ -tomy
6. ____ -tripsy
7. ____ -trophic

A. stopping
B. instrument for cutting
C. incision
D. forming of an opening
E. twitching
F. nutrition
G. surgical crushing

II. FILL IN THE BLANK.
Enter the correct word combination in the blank provided.

1. The combining form hem/o means blood. Hemo_____ would be the stopping of bleeding.

2. A _____ is the forming of an opening in the trachea (combining form trache/o).

3. An arteriotomy would be the _____ of an artery.

4. _____ means twitching.

5. If lith/o means stone, then lithotripsy is the _____ of a stone.

6. Hypertrophy is the overgrowth of an organ due to a kind of hyper_____.

7. An instrument used for cutting ends with _____.

III. TRUE/FALSE.
Mark the following true or false.

1. A craniotomy would be an incision of the cranium.
   ○ true
   ○ false

2. -Tome is an ending for an instrument for cutting.
   ○ true
   ○ false

3. If the combining form nephr/o refers to the kidney, then nephrostomy would be a closing of the kidney.

  ○ true
  ○ false

4. Atrophy is wasting away or a severe lack of nutrition.

  ○ true
  ○ false

5. Craniotomy means excision of the cranium.

  ○ true
  ○ false

Suffixes – Lesson 12 (Synonymous Suffixes)

In the prefixes unit we pointed out a few prefixes that have the same meanings. There are several suffixes which also present this problem. For example, the definition "condition" could correctly be assigned to the suffixes -osis, -ia, -iasis, AND -ism. In any instance where a definition is given that is appropriate for more than one suffix, one, both, or all suffixes would be correct. There will be some review exercises that require you to remember ALL suffixes with the same definition.

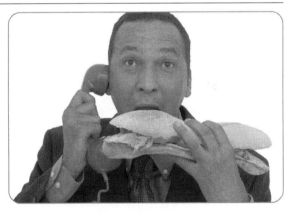

There are two suffixes that provide a peculiar problem when editing. These are -phagia and -phasia. Say these out loud. They sound exactly the same. While there are several word parts and words that create a similar problem for medical transcription editors, these are the only problem suffixes. It is important to note the differences and learn precisely which spelling means "speech" and which means "eating or swallowing." It is obvious that, while both deal with functions of the mouth, they have very different medical implications.

I. MATCHING.
Match the appropriate terms below.

1. ____ -ectomy
2. ____ -algia
3. ____ -gram
4. ____ -megaly
5. ____ -pathy
6. ____ -tripsy
7. ____ -emesis
8. ____ -meter
9. ____ -rrhea
10. ____ -logist
11. ____ -phagia
12. ____ -tomy
13. ____ -cele
14. ____ -phasia
15. ____ -centesis
16. ____ -scopy
17. ____ -ectasia
18. ____ -plasty
19. ____ -sclerosis
20. ____ -oma
21. ____ -rrhage
22. ____ -stasis
23. ____ -itis
24. ____ -malacia
25. ____ -ac

A. enlargement
B. vomiting
C. tumor
D. pertaining to
E. flow/discharge
F. a record
G. stopping
H. surgical crushing
I. incision
J. instrument to measure
K. specialist
L. procedure to aspirate fluid
M. speech
N. protrusion of an organ through its containing wall
O. pain
P. disease
Q. swallowing
R. examination with an instrument
S. dilation
T. surgical repair
U. excessive flow or discharge
V. inflammation
W. softening
X. excision or removal
Y. hardening

II. FILL IN THE BLANK.
Using the terms in the box, enter the correct word combination in the space provided.

1. Enter a word for removal of the appendix (combining form append/i). _____

2. Aphasia is inability to _____ .

3. Chondromalacia is _____ of the cartilage.

4. Enter a word that means enlargement of the liver (combining form hepat/o). _____

5. Hypokinesia is retarded, or below normal _____ .

6. Lithotripsy is _____ of a stone.

7. Hyperemesis is excessive _____ .

8. Mammoplasty is _____ of the breasts.

9. Amniocentesis is a procedure to _____ .

10. Osteopenia means _____ of bone.

11. Adenopathy is _____ of the adenoid tissue.

12. A specialist is _____ specializes.

13. A flexible sigmoidoscopy is an _____ of the sigmoid colon.

14. Cryogenic is the _____ of cold temperatures.

appendectomy
aspirate amniotic fluid
deficiency
disease
examination with an instrument
hepatomegaly
movement
one who
production
softening
speak
surgical crushing
surgical repair
vomiting

III. MULTIPLE CHOICE.
Choose the correct answer.

1. Kleptomania is (◯preoccupation with, ◯abnormal fear of, ◯capable of) stealing.

2. -Trophy means (◯surgical crushing, ◯nutrition, ◯enzyme).

3. (◯-Emia, ◯-Emesis, ◯-Edema) means swelling.

4. Dysphagia is difficulty (◯swallowing, ◯speaking, ◯seeing).

5. Dysphasia is difficulty (◯swallowing, ◯speaking, ◯seeing).

6. Which of the following is NOT a suffix that creates an adjective? ($\bigcirc$-ible, $\bigcirc$-al, $\bigcirc$-lysis).

7. The forming of an opening is ($\bigcirc$-tomy, $\bigcirc$-stomy, $\bigcirc$-cele).

IV. TRUE/FALSE.
Mark the following true or false.

1. -Logy is a specialist.
   $\bigcirc$ true
   $\bigcirc$ false

2. Hydrocele is a water hernia.
   $\bigcirc$ true
   $\bigcirc$ false

3. Amylase is a type of enzyme.
   $\bigcirc$ true
   $\bigcirc$ false

4. Lymphoma is a condition of the lymph nodes.
   $\bigcirc$ true
   $\bigcirc$ false

5. The suffix -pexy means surgical crushing.
   $\bigcirc$ true
   $\bigcirc$ false

6. Electroencephalography is the process of recording brain activity.
   $\bigcirc$ true
   $\bigcirc$ false

7. Myalgia is inflammation of the muscles.
   $\bigcirc$ true
   $\bigcirc$ false

8. The suffix which means rupture is -rrhaphy.
   $\bigcirc$ true
   $\bigcirc$ false

Review: Lessons 10–12

I. MATCHING.
Match the appropriate terms below.

1. ____ -sclerosis
2. ____ -rrhexis
3. ____ -tripsy
4. ____ -tomy
5. ____ -scopy
6. ____ -stasis
7. ____ -rrhaphy
8. ____ -trophic
9. ____ -rrhea
10. ____ -spasm
11. ____ -tome
12. ____ -stomy

A. an instrument for cutting
B. stopping
C. flow or discharge
D. rupture
E. forming of an opening
F. nutrition
G. suture
H. hardening
I. twitching
J. incision
K. surgical crushing
L. examination with an instrument

II. MULTIPLE CHOICE.
Choose the correct answer.

1. An incision is indicated by (◯-stomy, ◯-tomy, ◯-scopy).

2. A (◯-tripsy, ◯-stomy, ◯-scopy) would crush or break up something.

3. (◯-Rrhea, ◯-Rrhexis, ◯-Rrhaphy) means rupture.

III. FILL IN THE BLANK.
Using the terms in the box, enter the correct term(s) in the space provided.

1. An ileostomy would be the forming of a/an _____ in the ileum.

2. Bronchospasm is a/an _____ of the bronchus.

3. A capsulorrhaphy includes a/an _____ .

4. Flow or discharge is indicated by the suffix _____ .

5. An endoscopy is a/an _____ of some kind.

6. An osteotome is an instrument for _____ bone.

7. _____ is achieved when an increase is prevented.

cutting
examination
opening
rrhea
stasis
suture
twitching

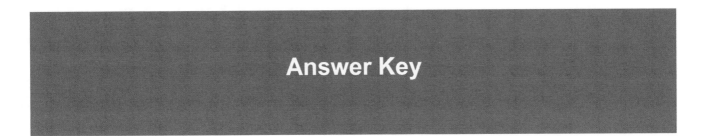

Answer Key

Word Building

Prefixes

I. FILL IN THE BLANK.

1. pre OR pre-
2. sub OR sub-
3. bi OR bi-
4. un OR un-
5. by OR by-
6. im OR im-
7. mid OR mid-
8. dis OR dis-
9. trans OR trans-
10. pre OR pre-
11. mal OR mal-
12. non OR non-

Suffixes

I. FILL IN THE BLANK.

1. ion OR -ion
2. ment OR -ment
3. ary OR -ary
4. able OR -able
5. ly OR -ly
6. ous OR -ous
7. ful OR -ful
8. able OR -able
9. al OR -al
10. er OR -er

Combining Forms

I. FILL IN THE BLANK.

1. cystocele
2. amniocentesis
3. cholecystectomy
4. pathologist
5. bronchospasm
6. adenopathy
7. jejunostomy
8. ophthalmic
9. cervicitis
10. salpingectomy
11. colostomy
12. thoracolumbar

Identifying Word Parts

I. MATCHING.

1. B. The main body or foundation of a word.
2. D. Syllable(s) placed at the front of a word to modify or change the meaning of the word.
3. C. Syllable(s) placed at the end of a word to modify or change the meaning of the word.
4. A. A root word plus a vowel.

II. FILL IN THE BLANK.

1. hydrosalpinx
2. cholecystectomy
3. organomegaly
4. hysterosalpingogram
5. choledochojejunostomy
6. esophagogastroduodenoscopy
7. endoscopy
8. lymphadenectomy
9. appendicitis
10. lumbosacral

Root Words

Root Words – Lesson 1 (Ab–Ad)

II. MATCHING.
1. C. extremities
3. D. abdomen
5. E. adenoids

2. B. gland
4. A. fat

III. SPELLING.
1. adenoidectomy
3. abdominal
5. adenocarcinoma

2. adipose
4. acromegaly

Root Words – Lesson 2 (Ae–Am)

II. MATCHING.
1. D. albumin
3. C. starch
5. A. white

2. E. amnion
4. B. air

III. MULTIPLE CHOICE.
1. starch
3. amni/o
5. amnion

2. air
4. white

Root Words – Lesson 3 (An–Ap)

II. MATCHING.
1. C. aorta
3. D. anterior
5. B. vessel

2. E. appendix
4. A. crooked

III. SPELLING.
1. ankylosing
3. anterolateral
5. angiogram

2. appendicitis
4. aortic

Root Words – Lesson 4 (Ar–At)

II. MATCHING.
1. B. joint
3. C. imperfect
5. B. joint

2. D. yellow, fatty plaque
4. A. artery

III. TRUE/FALSE.
1. true
3. true
5. false

2. false
4. false

Review: Lessons 1–4

I. MATCHING.

1. H. gland
2. K. joint
3. S. anterior or before
4. J. air
5. L. crooked or fused
6. A. extremities
7. B. aorta
8. K. joint
9. P. amnion
10. D. abdomen
11. Q. vessel
12. G. white
13. I. starch
14. C. imperfect
15. M. appendix
16. R. adenoids
17. E. fat
18. N. albumin
19. O. artery
20. F. yellow, fatty plaque

II. MULTIPLE CHOICE.

1. angiectomy
2. appendectomy
3. arthroplasty
4. arteriogram
5. amylase
6. adenoidectomy
7. intra-abdominal
8. appendicitis
9. adipogenesis
10. aortotomy

Root Words – Lesson 5 (Au–Br)

II. MATCHING.

1. B. ear
2. E. eyelid
3. D. embryonic form
4. C. arm
5. A. bile

III. MULTIPLE CHOICE.

1. ear
2. eyelid
3. arm
4. blast/o
5. bile

Root Words – Lesson 6 (Br–Ca)

II. MATCHING.

1. B. cheek
2. D. calcium
3. E. bursa
4. A. short
5. C. windpipe

III. SPELLING.

1. bronchospasm
2. buccal
3. brachyesophagus
4. bursectomy
5. calcium

Root Words – Lesson 7 (Ca)

II. MATCHING.

1. D. heart
2. E. carpus
3. A. cancer
4. B. tail
5. C. heel

III. MISSING LETTERS.

1. carcinoma
2. cardiomyopathy
3. calcaneocuboid
4. carpometacarpal
5. carpal

Root Words – Lesson 8 (Ce–Ch)

II. MATCHING.

1. C. brain
2. D. green
3. B. head
4. E. neck
5. A. cecum

III. TRUE/FALSE.

1. false
2. true
3. false
4. false
5. true

Review: Lessons 5–8

I. MATCHING.

1. B. heart
2. S. cheek
3. N. tail
4. O. neck
5. H. embryonic form
6. K. bursa
7. D. carpus
8. E. brain
9. A. ear
10. C. eyelid
11. R. arm
12. P. heel
13. Q. green
14. I. cancerous
15. T. bile
16. J. calcium
17. M. short
18. F. head
19. L. windpipe
20. G. cecum

II. MULTIPLE CHOICE.

1. cephalocaudal
2. aural
3. atherosclerosis
4. buccal
5. bronchiectasis
6. blastoma
7. cecectomy
8. carcinoma
9. cerebromalacia
10. cervicobrachialgia

Root Words – Lesson 9 (Ch–Cl)

II. MATCHING.

1. B. cartilage
2. C. fetal covering
3. A. bile
4. E. gallbladder
5. D. clavicle

III. MULTIPLE CHOICE.

1. chori/o
2. clavicle
3. cartilage
4. gallbladder
5. bile

Root Words – Lesson 10 (Co–Cr)

II. MATCHING.

1. D. colon
2. C. rib
3. A. hollow/vagina
4. E. cranium/skull
5. B. coccyx

III. SPELLING.

1. colonoscopy
2. coccygeal
3. craniocervical
4. costovertebral
5. colporrhaphy

Root Words – Lesson 11 (Cr–Cy)

II. MATCHING.

1. C. skin
2. A. cyst, bladder
3. D. hide, conceal
4. B. cold
5. E. blue

III. FILL IN THE BLANK.

1. cold
2. skin
3. blue
4. crypt/o
5. cyst/o

Root Words – Lesson 12 (Cy–De)

II. MATCHING.

1. D. teeth
2. E. right
3. A. skin
4. C. cell
5. B. finger/toe

III. MULTIPLE CHOICE.

1. right
2. teeth
3. finger/toe
4. cell
5. skin

Review: Lessons 9–12

I. MATCHING.

1. C. skin
2. G. teeth
3. R. conceal
4. P. gallbladder
5. O. blue
6. B. finger/toe
7. N. bile
8. C. skin
9. J. cell
10. S. vagina
11. E. right
12. M. cranium/skull
13. A. fetal covering
14. Q. bladder
15. F. cold
16. L. clavicle
17. D. colon
18. K. rib
19. H. cartilage
20. I. coccyx

II. TRUE/FALSE.

1. true
2. false
3. false
4. true
5. false
6. true
7. false
8. false
9. true
10. false

Root Words – Lesson 13 (Di–Du)

II. MATCHING.

1. C. thirst
2. B. disc
3. D. distant from origin
4. A. directed toward/on the back
5. E. duodenum

III. MISSING LETTERS.

1. polydipsia
2. dorsal
3. discogenic
4. duodenal
5. distally

Root Words – Lesson 14 (Ec–Er)

II. MATCHING.

1. C. brain
2. B. sound
3. A. red
4. E. electricity
5. D. intestine

III. SPELLING.

1. enterocolitis
2. electrodermal
3. encephalomalacia
4. erythrocyte
5. echogram

Root Words – Lesson 15 (Es–Fi)

II. MATCHING.

1. C. esophagus
2. E. fiber
3. D. feeling
4. A. fetus
5. B. femur

III. TRUE/FALSE.

1. true
2. false
3. false
4. false
5. true

Root Words – Lesson 16 (Fi–Ge)

II. MATCHING.

1. C. forehead
2. E. genitals
3. D. fibula
4. A. stomach
5. B. milk

III. MULTIPLE CHOICE.

1. stomach
2. front
3. genitals
4. fibula
5. milk

Review: Lessons 13–16

I. MATCHING.

1. S. duodenum
2. Q. disc
3. N. fiber
4. E. brain
5. G. milk
6. I. Stomach
7. H. sound
8. P. genitals
9. O. red
10. M. fetus
11. C. far
12. D. thirst
13. J. electricity
14. A. forehead
15. R. directed toward/on the back
16. K. fibula
17. B. femur
18. F. intestine
19. T. feeling
20. L. esophagus

II. TRUE/FALSE.

1. false
2. true
3. true
4. false
5. true
6. false
7. true
8. false
9. true
10. true

Root Words – Lesson 17 (Ge–Gn)

II. MATCHING.

1. D. tongue
2. C. old
3. A. jaw
4. B. glomerulus
5. E. sugar

III. MISSING LETTERS.

1. glossotonsillar
2. geriatric
3. hyperglycemia
4. gnathodynia
5. glomerulonephritis

Root Words – Lesson 18 (Gr–Hi)

II. MATCHING.

1. C. female
2. D. liver
3. E. tissue
4. A. grain
5. B. blood

III. TRUE/FALSE.

1. true
2. false
3. false
4. true
5. true

Root Words – Lesson 19 (Ho–Il)

II. MATCHING.

1. B. water
2. E. uterus
3. D. ileum
4. A. common/same
5. C. humerus

III. UNSCRAMBLE.

1. homogeneous
2. hydrometer
3. humeral
4. ileocecal
5. hysterosalpingogram

Root Words – Lesson 20 (Il–Ir)

II. MATCHING.

1. C. ilium
2. E. colored circle
3. D. intestine
4. B. lowermost/below
5. A. immune

III. MULTIPLE CHOICE.

1. infer/o
2. iris
3. immun/o
4. intestin/o

Review: Lessons 17–20

I. MATCHING.

1. S. hip bone
2. Q. same
3. H. immune
4. P. tissue
5. E. small intestine
6. T. intestine
7. I. liver
8. R. humerus
9. M. uterus
10. N. tongue
11. O. water
12. D. lowermost/below
13. K. jaw
14. B. colored circle
15. G. female
16. L. glomerulus
17. C. sugar
18. A. old
19. F. grain
20. J. blood

II. SPELLING.

1. homogeneous OR homogenous
2. inferior
3. sacroiliac
4. iridectomy
5. hydrometer
6. geriatric
7. gynecology
8. gnathodynia
9. glomerulus
10. hepatomegaly

Root Words – Lesson 21 (Is–La)

II. MATCHING.

1. E. milk
2. D. tear/crying
3. B. lip
4. A. ischium
5. C. jejunum

III. FILL IN THE BLANK.

1. lip
2. ischi/o
3. milk
4. lacrim/o
5. jejunum

Root Words – Lesson 22 (La–Li)

II. MATCHING.

1. D. flank
2. B. side
3. E. larynx
4. C. white
5. A. tongue

III. MISSING LETTERS.

1. leukocyte
2. lingula
3. laryngeal
4. laparoscope
5. anterolateral

Root Words – Lesson 23 (Li–Ly)

II. MATCHING.

1. D. stone
2. C. fat
3. B. lymph
4. A. lower back
5. E. lobe

III. MULTIPLE CHOICE.

1. stone
2. lumb/o
3. lobe
4. lymph node(s)
5. fat

Root Words – Lesson 24 (Ma–Me)

II. MATCHING.

1. C. month
2. D. membrane
3. A. breast
4. E. middle
5. B. black

III. UNSCRAMBLE.

1. mediolateral
2. meningocele
3. melanotic
4. mammogram
5. mastectomy

Review: Lessons 21–24

I. MATCHING.

1. P. larynx
2. H. ischium
3. M. side
4. R. month
5. S. lip
6. Q. breast
7. I. milk
8. E. flank
9. N. lymph
10. C. jejunum
11. F. white
12. G. lower back
13. J. membrane
14. D. tear/crying
15. L. middle
16. T. fat
17. K. lobe
18. A. stone
19. B. tongue
20. O. black

II. TRUE/FALSE.

1. false
2. true
3. false
4. true
5. true
6. false
7. false
8. true
9. true
10. true

Root Words – Lesson 25 (Me–My)

II. MATCHING.

1. C. muscle
2. D. uterine tissue
3. A. one
4. C. muscle
5. B. mucus

III. MISSING LETTERS.

1. mucoperiosteal
2. monoclonal
3. endometritis
4. myometrium
5. musculotendinous

Root Words – Lesson 26 (My–Ne)

II. MATCHING.

1. C. marrow
2. D. fungus
3. E. sleep
4. A. nose
5. B. new

III. TRUE/FALSE.

1. false
2. false
3. true
4. true
5. true

Root Words – Lesson 27 (Ne–Od)

II. MATCHING.

1. C. kidney
2. D. teeth
3. E. pain
4. A. nerve
5. B. dead

III. FILL IN THE BLANK.

1. kidney
2. odyn/o
3. teeth
4. Neur/o
5. necr/o

Root Words – Lesson 28 (On–Or)

II. MATCHING.

1. D. testicle
2. A. ovary
3. E. tumor
4. B. mouth
5. C. eye

III. UNSCRAMBLE.

1. oncology
2. intraoral
3. ophthalmology
4. orchiectomy
5. oophorosalpingitis

Review: Lessons 25–28

I. MATCHING.

1. I. mouth
2. L. new
3. B. marrow/spinal cord
4. G. tumor
5. H. testicle
6. E. sleep
7. D. uterine tissue
8. A. only
9. N. nose
10. O. nerve
11. M. eye
12. J. teeth
13. C. ovary
14. P. pain
15. Q. kidney
16. F. mucus
17. K. dead
18. S. muscle
19. S. muscle
20. R. fungus

II. MULTIPLE CHOICE.

1. neur/o
2. Ne/o
3. narc/o
4. or/o
5. orchi/o
6. Ophthalm/o
7. mon/o
8. My/o
9. metr/i
10. muscle

Root Words – Lesson 29 (Or–Pa)

II. MATCHING.

1. D. straight
2. E. kneecap
3. A. ear
4. B. bone
5. C. pancreas

III. TRUE/FALSE.

1. false
2. false
3. false
4. true
5. true

Root Words – Lesson 30 (Pa–Ph)

II. MATCHING.

1. E. pelvis
2. C. pharynx
3. D. peritoneum
4. A. disease
5. B. drugs

III. SPELLING.

1. intraperitoneal
2. pathologist
3. pelvimetry
4. cricopharyngeal
5. pharmacological

Root Words – Lesson 31 (Ph–Pl)

II. MATCHING.

1. E. light
2. D. pleura
3. A. vein
4. C. diaphragm
5. B. sound

III. UNSCRAMBLE.

1. phonation
2. costophrenic
3. pleurodesis
4. photophobia
5. phlebolith

Root Words – Lesson 32 (Po–Pr)

II. MATCHING.

1. B. breathing
2. E. nearest to the point of origin
3. D. toward the back
4. A. prostate
5. C. anus

III. MISSING LETTERS.

1. proximal
2. proctitis
3. prostatectomy
4. pneumothorax
5. posterolateral

Review: Lessons 29–32

I. MATCHING.

1. D. ear
2. K. prostate
3. E. bone
4. A. air/breathing
5. C. rectum
6. J. pelvis
7. F. nearest point of origin
8. N. peritoneum
9. M. straight
10. B. pharynx
11. H. disease
12. G. kneecap
13. S. toward the back
14. P. vein
15. O. pleura
16. R. light
17. T. diaphragm
18. Q. sound
19. L. pancreas
20. I. drugs

II. MULTIPLE CHOICE.

1. pneum/o
2. light
3. diaphragm
4. proct/o
5. sound
6. phleb/o
7. disease
8. pelv/i
9. oste/o
10. kneecap

Root Words – Lesson 33 (Ps–Py)

II. MATCHING.

1. D. pus
2. C. mind
3. E. pubis
4. A. false
5. B. lung

III. TRUE/FALSE.

1. false
2. false
3. false
4. true
5. true

Root Words – Lesson 34 (Py–Rh)

II. MATCHING.

1. D. kidneys
2. E. trough/renal pelvis
3. A. nose
4. B. rectum
5. C. radiant energy/radius

III. FILL IN THE BLANK.

1. ren/o
2. rhin/o
3. rectum
4. Pyel/o
5. Radi/o

Root Words – Lesson 35 (Sa–Se)

II. MATCHING.

1. C. sacrum
2. A. scrotum
3. D. semen
4. E. serum
5. B. tube

III. TRUE/FALSE.

1. false
2. true
3. true
4. true
5. false

Root Words – Lesson 36 (So–Sp)

II. MATCHING.

1. C. wedge
2. D. spleen
3. A. body
4. E. seed
5. B. sound

III. MISSING LETTERS.

1. spermatocele
2. somatization
3. hepatosplenomegaly
4. sphenoethmoid
5. sonogram

Review: Lessons 33–36

I. MATCHING.

1. O. rectum
2. H. spleen
3. N. sound
4. T. sacrum
5. J. pubis
6. D. wedge
7. I. nose
8. F. mind
9. C. pus
10. G. scrotum
11. L. seed
12. B. kidneys
13. S. lung
14. A. false
15. K. tube
16. R. body
17. P. serum
18. Q. semen
19. M. renal pelvis
20. E. radius

II. MULTIPLE CHOICE.

1. wedge
2. radiant energy
3. trough
4. mind
5. lung
6. somat/o
7. seed
8. pub/o
9. py/o

Root Words – Lesson 37 (Sp–Te)

II. MATCHING.

1. E. tendon
2. D. temple
3. B. sternum
4. A. vertebra
5. C. ankle bone

III. UNSCRAMBLE.

1. metatarsal
2. temporomandibular
3. spondylolisthesis
4. tenosynovitis
5. sternocleidomastoid

Root Words – Lesson 38 (Th–To)

II. MATCHING.

1. E. heat
2. D. tonsil
3. A. chest
4. B. lump/clot
5. C. tibia

III. TRUE/FALSE.

1. true
2. false
3. false
4. false
5. false

Root Words – Lesson 39 (To–Ur)

II. MATCHING.

1. D. ureter
2. E. ulna
3. A. urine
4. C. poison
5. B. windpipe

III. FILL IN THE BLANK.

1. ur/o
2. ureter/o
3. windpipe
4. Uln/o
5. poison

Root Words – Lesson 40 (Ur–Ve)

II. MATCHING.

1. E. urethra
2. D. uterus
3. C. vagus nerve
4. B. vessel
5. A. vein

III. MISSING LETTERS.

1. uterovaginal
2. vasovagal
3. urethritis
4. venotomy
5. vagotomy

Root Words – Lesson 41 (Ve–Xa)

II. MATCHING.

1. D. vulva
2. C. yellow
3. A. vertebra
4. B. belly side

III. TRUE/FALSE.

1. false
2. false
3. false
4. true
5. false

Review: Lessons 37–41

I. MATCHING.

1. U. urine
2. P. ankle bone
3. M. yellow
4. E. urethra
5. Q. sternum
6. K. tibia
7. B. vein
8. N. tonsil
9. G. vertebra
10. R. poison
11. L. belly side
12. T. vessel
13. H. vulva
14. A. heat
15. J. vagus nerve
16. V. tendon
17. S. ureter
18. F. temple
19. I. clot/thrombus
20. G. vertebra
21. W. trachea
22. C. ulna
23. D. chest
24. O. uterus

II. MULTIPLE CHOICE.

1. trache/o
2. thrombus
3. ankle bone
4. temple
5. tonsil
6. ulna
7. vessel
8. yellow
9. belly side
10. ven/o

Prefixes

Prefixes – Lesson 1 (A)

I. MATCHING.

1. E. against
2. D. away from
3. A. without
4. C. before
5. B. toward

II. MULTIPLE CHOICE.

1. away from
2. ante-
3. against
4. a-
5. toward

III. FILL IN THE BLANK.
1. anemia
2. ad- OR ad
3. ab- OR ab
4. contra- OR contra
5. antenatal

Prefixes – Lesson 2 (Bi–Dy)

I. MATCHING.
1. C. difficult
2. A. down from
3. D. two
4. E. across
5. B. slow

II. TRUE/FALSE.
1. false
2. true
3. false
4. false
5. true

III. FILL IN THE BLANK.
1. dyspepsia
2. bimanual
3. dehydration
4. bradycardia
5. through

Prefixes – Lesson 3 (Ec–He)

I. MATCHING.
1. C. half
2. E. without/outside
3. A. above
4. B. good
5. D. inside

II. TRUE/FALSE.
1. false
2. true
3. false
4. false
5. true

III. FILL IN THE BLANK.
1. eumenorrhea
2. epidural
3. exhale
4. half
5. endocardial

Review: Lessons 1–3

I. MATCHING.
1. C. against
2. E. difficult
3. H. half
4. B. no
5. K. removing
6. I. without/outside
7. M. through
8. A. toward
9. N. good
10. F. two
11. G. inside
12. J. away from
13. L. on
14. O. before
15. D. slow

II. TRUE/FALSE.

1. false
2. true
3. false
4. true
5. false
6. true

III. MULTIPLE CHOICE.

1. antihypertensive
2. bradyarrhythmia
3. asymmetry
4. decompression
5. half
6. two
7. difficulty
8. euthanasia
9. through

IV. FILL IN THE BLANK.

1. bifocal
2. dia- OR dia
3. epitrochlear
4. endometritis
5. decongestant
6. prenatal OR antenatal
7. anti-inflammatory OR antiinflammatory
8. dysphasia
9. toward
10. away from
11. hemilaminectomy
12. anesthesia
13. epi OR epi-
14. eupnea
15. bradyarrhythmia

Prefixes – Lesson 4 (Hy–In)

I. MATCHING.

1. E. not
2. D. beneath, C. below normal OR C
3. D. beneath
4. A. excessive
5. B. between

II. MULTIPLE CHOICE.

1. hypercholesterolemia
2. hypoglossal
3. not
4. Infra-
5. intervertebral

III. FILL IN THE BLANK.

1. inter- OR inter
2. beneath OR below
3. Hyperactivity
4. inactive
5. hypoglycemia

Prefixes – Lesson 5 (In–Mi)

I. MATCHING.

1. A. large
2. E. middle
3. B. within
4. C. bad
5. D. small

II. MULTIPLE CHOICE.

1. malalignment
2. inside
3. small
4. large
5. meso-

III. FILL IN THE BLANK.

1. microembolus
2. within OR inside of
3. malrotation
4. middle
5. large

Prefixes – Lesson 6 (Mu–Pe)

I. MATCHING.
1. E. one
2. B. through
3. A. many
4. C. none
5. D. near

II. TRUE/FALSE.
1. true
2. false
3. true
4. false
5. false

III. FILL IN THE BLANK.
1. through
2. para-appendicitis OR peri-appendicitis
3. polydipsia
4. unipolar OR monopolar
5. nonei- OR nonei

Review: Lessons 4–6

I. MATCHING.
1. A. within
2. E. bad
3. B. excessive
4. C. many
5. L. small
6. M. through
7. D. not
8. I. large
9. K. none
10. F. beside
11. G. below normal
12. H. one
13. J. beneath (positionally)
14. N. middle
15. O. between

II. MULTIPLE CHOICE.
1. beneath
2. multi-
3. within
4. through
5. smallness
6. one
7. hyper-
8. intercartilaginous

III. FILL IN THE BLANK.
1. hyperpnea
2. through
3. intracranial
4. multilobular OR multilobar
5. nonei- OR nonei
6. mesothelial
7. malabsorption
8. one
9. infraorbital
10. parahepatic
11. small
12. insubstantial
13. between
14. large
15. subdiaphragmatic OR infradiaphragmatic

IV. TRUE/FALSE.
1. false
2. false
3. false
4. true
5. true
6. false
7. true

Prefixes – Lesson 7 (Pe–Re)

I. MATCHING.
1. A. after
3. D. around
5. B. first

2. E. again
4. C. backward

II. MULTIPLE CHOICE.
1. around
3. behind
5. first

2. again
4. Post-

III. FILL IN THE BLANK.
1. behind/backward OR behind
3. first
5. again

2. peritonsillar
4. after

Prefixes – Lesson 8 (Su–Un)

I. MATCHING.
1. C. fast
3. E. one
5. B. together

2. D. across
4. F. above
6. A. excessive

II. TRUE/FALSE.
1. true
3. true
5. true

2. false
4. false
6. false

III. FILL IN THE BLANK.
1. uni- OR uni
3. tachy- OR tachy
5. above OR over

2. union
4. across/through OR across
6. super- OR super

Prefixes – Lesson 10 (Synonymous Prefixes)

I. MATCHING.
1. B. large
3. D. around
5. G. half, partly
7. K. out/without/outside
9. M. bad
11. I. fast
13. Q. against
15. H. slow
17. A. backward
19. E. first

2. J. difficult
4. T. between
6. F. toward
8. L. within
10. P. excessive
12. S. near, beside
14. N. away from
16. R. middle
18. O. after
20. C. above, over

II. MULTIPLE ANSWER.
1. para-, dys-
3. epi-, supra-

2. hypo-, sub-, infra-
4. inter-, dia-

III. MULTIPLE CHOICE.

1. per- OR per
2. brady- OR brady
3. nonei- OR nonei
4. endo- OR endo
5. post- OR post
6. hemi- OR hemi

IV. TRUE/FALSE.

1. true
2. false
3. false
4. true
5. true

Review: Lessons 7–10

I. MATCHING.

1. G. around
2. L. beside
3. B. union
4. K. fast
5. J. between
6. M. one
7. I. above
8. C. excessive
9. A. after
10. H. again
11. E. within
12. D. backward
13. F. first
14. N. below normal

II. MULTIPLE CHOICE.

1. hypo-
2. hyper-
3. intra-
4. hypo-
5. inter-
6. fast
7. primipara
8. Re-
9. backward
10. behind
11. one

Suffixes

Suffixes – Lesson 1 (Ab–Ce)

I. MULTIPLE CHOICE.

1. noun
2. adjective
3. adjective
4. noun
5. adjective
6. adjective
7. noun
8. adjective
9. adjective
10. adjective

II. MATCHING.

1. C. hernia
2. D. pain
3. A. enzyme
4. E. pertaining to
5. B. capable of

III. MULTIPLE CHOICE.

1. -cele
2. -ic OR -eal
3. -algia
4. -ible OR -able
5. -ase

IV. FILL IN THE BLANK.

1. compressible
2. arthralgia
3. enzyme
4. cystocele
5. appendiceal OR appendicular

Suffixes – Lesson 2 (Ce–Em)

I. MATCHING.

1. A. swelling
2. D. procedure to aspirate fluid
3. B. dilation
4. E. vomiting
5. C. excision or removal

II. MULTIPLE CHOICE.

1. -ectasia
2. -edema
3. -centesis
4. -ectomy
5. -emesis

III. FILL IN THE BLANK.

1. atelectasis OR atelectasia
2. appendectomy
3. hematemesis
4. amniocentesis
5. swelling

Suffixes – Lesson 3 (Em–Gr)

I. MATCHING.

1. E. instrument
2. C. blood
3. D. beginning
4. A. record
5. B. process of recording

II. MULTIPLE CHOICE.

1. -emia
2. -Genesis
3. -graph
4. -graphy
5. -gram

III. FILL IN THE BLANK.

1. blood
2. cardiogram
3. cardiography
4. cardiograph
5. osteogenesis

Review: Lessons 1–3

I. MATCHING.

1. L. procedure to aspirate fluid
2. F. enzyme
3. I. dilation
4. H. pain
5. M. blood
6. O. instrument for recording
7. N. excision or removal
8. C. capable of
9. G. process of recording
10. B. swelling
11. D. beginning/production
12. K. record
13. A. hernia
14. E. vomiting
15. J. pertaining to

II. FILL IN THE BLANK.

1. amniocentesis
2. procedure to aspirate fluid
3. excision OR removal
4. dictionary
5. blood
6. rectocele
7. pain
8. hyperemesis
9. echocardiogram
10. enzyme
11. cryogenic

Suffixes – Lesson 4 (I)

I. MATCHING.

1. B. one who
2. A. condition
3. A. condition
4. A. condition
5. C. inflammation

II. MULTIPLE CHOICE.

1. -itis
2. -itis
3. -itis
4. -ist

III. TRUE/FALSE.

1. true
2. true
3. true
4. true

Suffixes – Lesson 5 (Ki–Ly)

I. MATCHING.

1. D. pertaining to destruction
2. E. movement/motion
3. B. loosening/freeing
4. A. study of
5. C. specialist

II. MULTIPLE CHOICE.

1. -logy
2. -lysis
3. -lysis
4. movement
5. pathologist

III. FILL IN THE BLANK.

1. dyskinesia OR dyskinesis
2. biology
3. spondylolysis
4. specializes

Suffixes – Lesson 6 (M)

I. MATCHING.

1. C. preoccupation
2. E. instrument to measure
3. A. enlargement
4. D. softening
5. B. process of measuring

II. FILL IN THE BLANK.

1. softening
2. process of measuring flow
3. enlargement
4. mania
5. meter

III. TRUE/FALSE.

1. false
2. true
3. true
4. true
5. false

Review: Lessons 4–6

I. MATCHING.

1. K. enlargement
2. B. process of measuring
3. D. condition
4. C. study of
5. M. one who
6. A. softening
7. L. loosening/breaking apart/freeing
8. G. movement/motion
9. D. condition
10. F. preoccupation
11. H. instrument to measure
12. E. pertaining to destruction
13. J. inflammation
14. I. specialist

II. FILL IN THE BLANK.

1. cardiology
2. meter OR oximeter
3. inflammation
4. condition
5. enlargement
6. mania
7. softening
8. specialist in urology OR one who studies urology
9. bradykinesia OR bradykinesis

Suffixes – Lesson 7 (Oi–Os)

I. MATCHING.

1. A. vision
2. E. resembling
3. D. condition
4. C. tumor
5. B. sugar

II. FILL IN THE BLANK.

1. vision
2. sugar
3. tumor
4. mucoid
5. condition

III. TRUE/FALSE.

1. false
2. true
3. true
4. false
5. true

Suffixes – Lesson 8 (Ou–Ph)

I. MATCHING.

1. D. deficiency
2. B. disease
3. A. eating/swallowing
4. C. pertaining to
5. E. surgical fixation

II. FILL IN THE BLANK.

1. swallowing OR eating
2. deficiency
3. adenomatous
4. surgical fixation
5. -pathy OR pathy

III. TRUE/FALSE.

1. true
2. false
3. true
4. true
5. false

Suffixes – Lesson 9 (Ph–Rr)

I. MATCHING.
1. C. excessive flow or discharge
2. A. speech
3. E. surgical repair
4. B. abnormal fear
5. D. paralysis

II. FILL IN THE BLANK.
1. aphasia
2. plasty
3. bleeding excessively
4. paralysis
5. abnormally fearful OR excessively fearful

III. TRUE/FALSE.
1. false
2. true
3. false
4. true
5. false

Review: Lessons 7–9

I. MATCHING.
1. K. condition
2. J. surgical fixation
3. M. eating/swallowing
4. G. surgical repair
5. F. deficiency
6. L. sugar
7. A. vision
8. B. speech
9. O. disease
10. I. tumor
11. C. excessive flow or discharge
12. D. resembling
13. H. paralysis
14. E. characterized by
15. N. abnormal fear

II. TRUE/FALSE.
1. true
2. false
3. true
4. false
5. false
6. true
7. true
8. false
9. false
10. true

Suffixes – Lesson 10 (Rr–Sc)

I. MATCHING.
1. B. rupture
2. E. examination with an instrument
3. D. hardening
4. C. suture
5. A. flow or discharge

II. FILL IN THE BLANK.
1. hardening
2. rupture
3. examined
4. instrument
5. herniorrhaphy
6. flow or discharge OR flow/discharge

III. TRUE/FALSE.
1. true
2. false
3. true
4. false
5. false

Suffixes – Lesson 11 (Sp–Tr)

I. MATCHING.

1. B. instrument for cutting
2. E. twitching
3. A. stopping
4. D. forming of an opening
5. C. incision
6. G. surgical crushing
7. F. nutrition

II. FILL IN THE BLANK.

1. stasis
2. tracheostomy
3. incision
4. spasm OR -spasm
5. surgical crushing
6. nutrition OR plasia
7. -tome OR tome

III. TRUE/FALSE.

1. true
2. true
3. false
4. true
5. false

Suffixes – Lesson 12 (Synonymous Suffixes)

I. MATCHING.

1. X. excision or removal
2. O. pain
3. F. a record
4. A. enlargement
5. P. disease
6. H. surgical crushing
7. B. vomiting
8. J. instrument to measure
9. E. flow/discharge
10. K. specialist
11. Q. swallowing
12. I. incision
13. N. protrusion of an organ through its containing wall
14. M. speech
15. L. procedure to aspirate fluid
16. R. examination with an instrument
17. S. dilation
18. T. surgical repair
19. Y. hardening
20. C. tumor
21. U. excessive flow or discharge
22. G. stopping
23. V. inflammation
24. W. softening
25. D. pertaining to

II. FILL IN THE BLANK.

1. appendectomy
2. speak
3. softening
4. hepatomegaly
5. movement OR motion
6. surgical crushing
7. vomiting
8. surgical repair
9. aspirate amniotic fluid
10. deficiency
11. disease
12. one who
13. examination with an instrument
14. production

III. MULTIPLE CHOICE.

1. preoccupation with
2. nutrition
3. -edema
4. swallowing
5. speaking
6. -lysis
7. -stomy OR stomy

IV. TRUE/FALSE.

1. false
2. true
3. true
4. false
5. false
6. true
7. false
8. false

Review: Lessons 10–12

I. MATCHING.

1. H. hardening
2. D. rupture
3. K. surgical crushing
4. J. incision
5. L. examination with an instrument
6. B. stopping
7. G. suture
8. F. nutrition
9. C. flow or discharge
10. I. Twitching
11. A. an instrument for cutting
12. E. forming of an opening

II. MULTIPLE CHOICE.

1. -tomy OR tomy
2. -tripsy OR tripsy
3. -rrhexis OR rrhexis

III. FILL IN THE BLANK.

1. opening
2. twitching
3. suture
4. -rrhea OR rrhea
5. examination
6. cutting
7. stasis

Medical Word Building

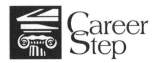

Career Step, LLC
Phone: 801.489.9393
Toll-Free: 800.246.7837
Fax: 801.491.6645
careerstep.com

This text companion contains a snapshot of the online program content converted to a printed format. Please note that the online training program is constantly changing and improving and is always the source of the most up-to-date information.

Product Number: HG-PR-11-001
Generation Date: February 2, 2012

Table of Contents